B
01
47
968

37547

PERGAMON INTERNATIONAL
POPULAR SCIENCE SERIES

THE ORIGIN OF THE SOLAR SYSTEM

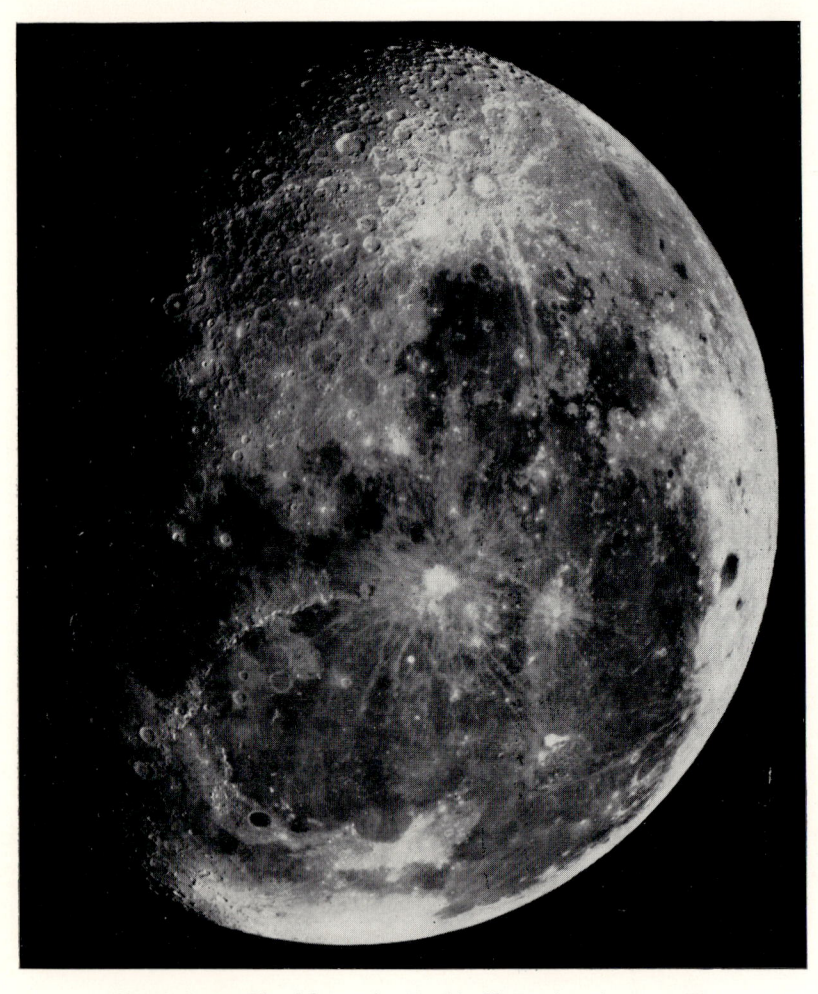

(*Frontispiece*). The Moon, the Earth's illustrative giant satellite, heavily bombarded, but also showing spontaneous volcanism. The main circular grey field is Mare Imbrium.

THE ORIGIN OF THE SOLAR SYSTEM

BY

H. P. BERLAGE

*Formerly of the Royal Netherlands Meteorological
Institute, De Bilt, and University of Utrecht, Netherlands*

PERGAMON PRESS

OXFORD · LONDON · EDINBURGH · NEW YORK
TORONTO · SYDNEY · PARIS · BRAUNSCHWEIG

PERGAMON PRESS LTD.,
Headington Hill Hall, Oxford
4 & 5 Fitzroy Square, London W.1

PERGAMON PRESS (SCOTLAND) LTD.,
2 & 3 Teviot Place, Edinburgh 1

PERGAMON PRESS INC.,
44–01 21st Street, Long Island City, New York 11101

PERGAMON OF CANADA LTD.,
207 Queen's Quay West, Toronto 1

PERGAMON PRESS (AUST.) PTY. LTD.,
Rushcutters Bay, Sydney, New South Wales

PERGAMON PRESS S.A.R.L.,
24 rue des Écoles, Paris 5e

VIEWEG & SOHN GmbH,
Burgplatz 1, Braunschweig

Copyright © 1968 Pergamon Press Ltd.
First Edition 1968 PERGAMON INTERNATIONAL
POPULAR SCIENCE SERIES
Library of Congress Catalog Card No. 67–31500

Printed in Great Britain by A. Wheaton & Co., Exeter

This book is sold subject to the condition
that it shall not, by way of trade, be lent,
resold, hired out, or otherwise disposed
of without the publisher's consent,
in any form of binding or cover
other than that in which
it is published.

08 003676 7 (flexicover)
08 003865 4 (hard cover)

Contents

		Page
1.	Introduction	1
2.	The structure of the planetary system	2
3.	The difficulty of the problem of planetary evolution	7
4.	Satellite systems small-scale copies of the planetary system	8
5.	Great scientists in the past on the right track	10
6.	Tidal forces	12
7.	Does the primeval nebula suffer local condensation?	13
8.	Laplace's theory	14
9.	Concentric rings	16
10.	The position of the axes of rotation of the planets	16
11.	Gas rings round a star possible	18
12.	The Trojans	18
13.	The flat disk archetype	20
14.	The dualistic conception of the solar system	21
15.	The tidal theory in its original form	22
16.	The tidal theory in its final form	23
17.	The gain obtained by tidal interaction	25
18.	Is the planetary system unique?	26
19.	The expanding universe	26
20.	Was it a catastrophe at the start?	27
21.	Did a resisting medium do the job?	28
22.	The theories of Lyttleton and Hoyle	29
23.	The hypothesis of Dauvillier	31
24.	Did electric forces enter the scene?	33

		Page
25.	A good start is half the work (Dutch proverb)	34
26.	The internal friction of the gas	35
27.	The theorem of minimum loss of energy due to viscosity in steady motion	35
28.	Steady conditions associated with non-uniform axial rotation	36
29.	Tendencies in the primeval nebula	37
30.	Dispersion of the primeval nebula	39
31.	The primeval nebula—was it turbulent?	40
32.	Local condensations caused by turbulence	47
33.	The different chemical composition of the planets	48
34.	The primeval nebula of cosmic composition	50
35.	When did the primeval nebula lose its hydrogen and helium?	51
36.	Temperatures in the primeval nebula	54
37.	Gases, liquids, and solids in the primeval nebula	56
38.	Meteorites	57
39.	Comets	58
40.	Saturn's rings	59
41.	The theoretical structure of the solar nebula	61
42.	The solar nebula a Cartesian vortex as well as a Kantian disk	65
43.	From a Kantian disk to Laplacean rings	65
44.	Strong arguments for the ring phase	67
45.	Can we explain the rule of Titius and Bode?	69
46.	The masses of the planets to a first approximation	71
47.	The outer limit of the solar system	72
48.	Further adjustment of the theory and what results from this	73
49.	The mean densities of planets and satellites	75
50.	The chemical composition of planets and satellites	76

Contents vii

		Page
51.	Is there an unfinished or exploded planet between Mars and Jupiter?	80
52.	The coming and going of comets	80
53.	Is the ring of asteroids dispersed?	82
54.	Radiation pressure, Poynting–Robertson effect, and zodiacal light	83
55.	Large-scale turbulence again	85
56.	Is the "inversion" of the axial rotation of the protoplanets an effect of solar tidal forces?	86
57.	The process of condensation of planetary rings	89
58.	The planetesimal hypothesis is probably right	93
59.	The origin of satellites	95
60.	Nature prefers even numbers of satellites	95
61.	Dimensions and limits of satellite systems	96
62.	Retrograde satellites	98
63.	The two remaining great puzzles	99
64.	Earth and Moon	100
65.	Equilibrium figures of spinning liquid masses	104
66.	Did resonance produce the Moon?	107
67.	Was the Moon expelled from the Earth?	108
68.	Did the Earth capture the Moon?	110
69.	Was the Moon perhaps a normal satellite?	111
70.	Neptune and its satellites	113
71.	The question of Pluto	115
72.	The systems of Jupiter, Saturn, and Uranus as family portraits	117
73.	Comparative anatomy of all satellite systems	121
74.	Why not satellites of satellites?	124
75.	A few words about our home in the solar system	125
	Bibliography	127
	Author Index	129

1. Introduction

"Say first, of God above or man below,
What can we reason, but from what we know?"

(ALEXANDER POPE)

THE problem of the origin and evolution of the solar system has a long and interesting history. It has been discussed by many generations of the greatest scientists. Clearer and sounder theories are now emerging and this, in part, is due to the new data obtained from space probes.

It is always difficult to explain to the general reader work which is being done at the very frontiers of a science. On the one hand, bright journalistic writings and illustrations may simplify to such an extent as to give wrong impressions. On the other hand, a full academic discussion may give so much of both sides of all the arguments and present such a mass of information as to obscure the main outline of the subject. A French proverb tells us that "the art of being boring is to say everything".

The author decided to abstain from the popular style and even to use, when occasion demands, a mathematical formulation. The book will need some application and cannot be read as a bedside novel.

By dividing the book into a large number of short sections an attempt has been made to spotlight the arguments for and against the various hypotheses which have been advanced from time to time. The author has tried to adjudicate as fairly as he can and to lead the reader through the mass of often conflicting theories on this important subject.

It may possibly be felt that some serious suggestions have

been discarded too lightly. The author can assure the reader that all the evidence has been very carefully considered and that a very representative collection of all shades of opinion is presented in this book. The reader will rightly feel, when he concludes the perusal of this evidence, that we are, in fact, very near to a solution of this age-old problem.

2. The Structure of the Planetary System

THE centre of the planetary system is occupied by the Sun, a yellow star whose photosphere radiates at a temperature of 5800°C absolute. The Sun, although a star of minor weight, has a mass 330,000 times greater than the mass of the Earth; it is even 740 times greater than the total mass of the planets. The Sun is a gaseous sphere of mean density 1·41. This average value leaves us in doubt about how the density in the solar globe increases from the surface to the centre. However, it is important to know that the Sun is a star, specifically heavier, but not much heavier, than water.

Around the Sun a series of planets circulate (Fig. 1). In succession from the centre towards the periphery of the system these planets are: Mercury, Venus, Earth, Mars, Jupiter, Saturn, Uranus, Neptune, and Pluto. Between Mars and Jupiter we meet a swarm of very small planets. These little planets are called "asteroids" in current British and American literature. They should be called "planetoids", as they were in the early days of their discovery. The term asteroid would suggest a little star rather than a little planet.

There is an essential difference in structure between a star and a planet. Stars are celestial bodies of large mass, gaseous, and spontaneous sources of radiation. Planets are bodies of smaller mass and are more or less cold globes. The light which makes them visible is reflected sunlight.

The Structure of the Planetary System

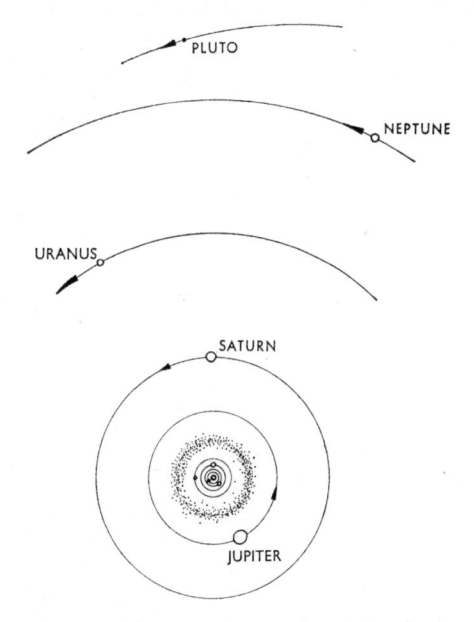

FIG. 1. The planetary system viewed from the north. The radii of the orbits of the planets only are given in the right proportions.

The word "circulate" for the motion of the planets round the Sun is to the point. The planetary orbits are in fact ellipses, but their "eccentricities" are small (Table 1). The innermost

TABLE 1. ECCENTRICITIES OF PLANETARY ORBITS

Mercury	0·206
Venus	0·007
Earth	0·017
Mars	0·093
Jupiter	0·048
Saturn	0·056
Uranus	0·046
Neptune	0·009
Pluto	0·246

planet, Mercury, and the outermost planet, Pluto, are the only ones moving in outstandingly eccentric orbits. During the passage through its "perihelion", Pluto comes slightly nearer to the Sun than does Neptune.

Another characteristic of the solar system is the near coincidence of the orbital planes of the planets. If the Earth's orbital plane, the "ecliptic", is used as a plane of reference; the inclinations of the orbits of the planets are those given in Table 2.

TABLE 2. INCLINATIONS OF PLANETARY ORBITS TO THE ECLIPTIC

Mercury	7° 0′
Venus	3° 24′
Earth	0
Mars	1° 51′
Jupiter	1° 19′
Saturn	2° 30′
Uranus	9° 46′
Neptune	1° 47′
Pluto	17° 19′

It is equally remarkable that the planets all move around the Sun in one and the same sense, counterclockwise when viewed from the north. This sense is designated as the "direct" sense. The Sun rotates in the direct sense about an axis inclined by no more than 5° to the normal to the ecliptic.

Moreover, and this is without any doubt the most spectacular property of the solar system, the orbits of the planets have not random dimensions. The average distances of the planets from the Sun fit a certain rule. It was described by Kepler (1571–1630) as the "harmony of the spheres". Titius, a Wittenberg mathematician, and Bode, a Berlin astronomer, gave it in 1772 the following form. If 0·4 is added to each term of the geometric series 0, 0·3, 0·6, 1·2, 2·4, 4·8, 9·6, 19·2, we obtain the series of the radii of the planetary orbits, expressed with reference to the mean radius of the Earth's orbit as the basic unit. This unit is known as the astronomical unit (a.u.).

Now, strictly speaking, zero is not the first term of the above geometric series. If this small defect is overlooked, the agreement between the theoretical and actual distances of the planets from the Sun is surprisingly close. This is confirmed by Table 3.

TABLE 3. APPROXIMATION OF THE RADII OF THE PLANETARY ORBITS (1) BY TITIUS'S AND BODE'S RULE (2) AND BY GEOMETRIC PROGRESSION (3)

	(1)	(2)	(3)
Mercury	0·39	0·4	0·32
Venus	0·72	0·7	0·56
Earth	1	1	1
Mars	1·52	1·6	1·77
Asteroids		2·8	3·13
Jupiter	5·20	5·2	5·55
Saturn	9·55	10·0	9·82
Uranus	19·22	19·6	17·37
Neptune	30·1	38·8	30·75

Evidently, the swarm of asteroids has taken the place of one of the planets. Moreover, in Titius's and Bode's time Neptune and Pluto were still unknown planets. Neptune was discovered in 1846, Pluto not until 1930. These two peripheral planets do not conform to Titius's and Bode's rule. For Neptune this rule leads to 38·8, whereas Neptune circulates at an average distance of 30·1 a.u. from the Sun. For Pluto the rule forecasts 77·2, whereas Pluto's average distance from the Sun amounts actually to no more than 39·4 a.u. Moreover, Pluto moves in a rather strongly inclined elliptic orbit and consequently may well be considered as a stray body.

Disregarding Pluto for a moment, and noting the relative smallness of the additive constant 0·4 applied in the above rule, we may say that Table 3 shows how far this approximation goes if the constant is chosen to be 1·77. The radii of the planetary orbits follow a geometric series. Hence, if r_{n+1} and r_n denote the radii of the orbits of two successive planets,

$$r_{n+1} : r_n = \text{constant}. \tag{1}$$

In any case, the actual series, be it represented by whatever formula, is so regular that any cosmogony failing to take it into account would be unacceptable.

One feature of the planetary system still requiring our attention is the mode of rotation of the planets and the obliquity of their axes. Mercury and Venus direct apparently one and the same hemisphere toward the Sun, although not as rigidly as the Moon does with respect to the Earth. As regards Venus (Plate I), the most probable state, according to recent radar observations, is an axial rotation slightly slower than its revolution round the Sun. On the other hand, there are indications that the period of rotation of the eccentric Mercury is decidedly shorter than the duration of its revolution round the Sun.

Pluto's axial rotation is still unknown. The other planets, as is shown by Table 4, spin around axes clearly tending to a position perpendicular to their orbital planes. The case of

TABLE 4. INCLINATIONS OF AXIS OF ROTATION OF THE PLANETS TO THEIR ORBITAL PLANES

Mercury	—
Venus	—
Earth	66° 33'
Mars	64° 48'
Jupiter	86° 54'
Saturn	63° 16'
Uranus	8° —
Neptune	61° —
Pluto	—

Uranus is unique. The axis of rotation of Uranus is nearly coincident with this planet's orbital plane. The near perpendicular position of the axes of the other planets is associated with a rotation in the direct sense.

In order to complete our elementary sketch of the solar system, it is instructive to review the masses of the planets. They are contained in Table 5. Pluto's mass is not yet accurately

TABLE 5. THE MASSES OF THE PLANETS EXPRESSED IN EARTH-MASSES

Mercury	0·054
Venus	0·814
Earth	1
Mars	0·107
Jupiter	317·5
Saturn	95·1
Uranus	14·5
Neptune	17·2
Pluto	0·05 ?

known. The value given here is considered to be the most probable. If the planet's density is about 3, this mass would agree with Kuiper's observations of the planet's diameter, but, curiously enough, it is then too small to be responsible for the perturbations in the motions of Uranus and Neptune which led to Pluto's discovery.

3. The Difficulty of the Problem of Planetary Evolution

EVEN when we exclude all satellites from our picture of the solar system, we are fascinated by the stringency of the rules which it obeys. The solar system is of almost crystalline structure. It is one of the most prominent examples of the natural evolution of disorder to order. We are aware of a creative force in the planetary system, just as we are aware of the hand of the potter in a porcelain vase.

The basic reason why the problem of the origin and evolution of the solar system eluded us for centuries is this: that no second example of such a system is known to us. Even the most thorough scanning of the sky with our present-day magnificent telescopes has never revealed other families of planets. Planets radiate too weakly in comparison with their mother star. There are, it is true, some stars subjected to periodic shifts, indicating the existence of a companion of much smaller mass, moving round the major one, but even in these cases we are far from the mass ratios that exist between the primaries and secondaries in our system. If the development of eclipsing binaries and close double stars were a process related to the development of planetary systems, we could point to hundreds of such pairs in different phases of evolution. But as regards planetary systems, we meet only our own.

Our planetary system might be unique in the literal sense; a quite exceptional creature, a pathological case. This possibility should be weighed seriously. On the other hand, such extreme individuality seems improbable. The number of double stars is estimated to be about half the total number of stars, and wherever a double star is born there is no home for planets. But why, among millions of millions of apparently singular stars, should there not be a large number carrying a wreath of planets?

We are acquainted with only one example and it is practically finished. Consequently, the history of our planetary system is a fully open question. Where do we find the materials on which to base an answer to this question? May scientists today cherish any more hope of finding a solution than the many generations of astronomers who have wrestled with the problem in the past?

4. Satellite Systems Small-scale Copies of the Planetary System

FORTUNATELY, our statement about being acquainted with only one planetary system is not strictly true. The Earth has one satellite—the Moon. Mars and Neptune have two satellites, Uranus has five, Jupiter twelve, and Saturn ten satellites and a set of rings. Saturn's system is shown in Fig. 2. When the peripheral "retrograde" satellites—those circulating round their planet in a direction contrary to the normal direction— are left out of account for the moment, the secondary systems of Jupiter and Saturn show surprisingly intimate relations with the primary system.

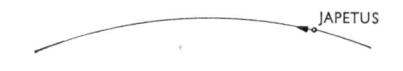

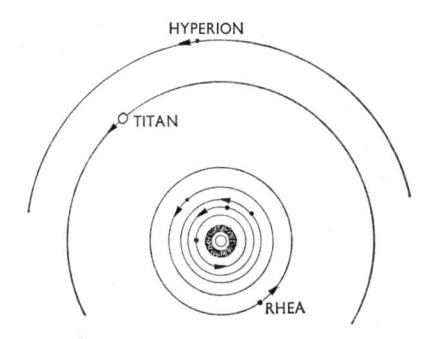

FIG. 2. The satellite system of Saturn, a small-scale replica of the planetary system. The retrograde satellite Phoebe is outside the figure.

The secondary systems and the primary system must have been created in the same way. No theory of the origin of the solar system, failing to explain the evolution of the secondary systems as elegantly as the evolution of the primary system, is acceptable.

5. Great Scientists in the Past on the Right Track

WHEN surveying physical studies in modern times, as a rule it seems irrelevant to go through the history of a question and the answers given, because the answers given at present differ in essence from those given in the past, even from those appearing reasonable in the very recent past. Theories such as those of relativity, of elementary particles, of electromagnetic fields and cosmic plasma, as well as the electronic resources that have come to our assistance, have revolutionized physical sciences to such an extent that hypotheses dating from before the twentieth century are often hopelessly antiquated. What makes the study of the origin and development of the solar system so fascinating is just the reverse. Several great thinkers, in the course of over three centuries, have lifted tips of the veil that has remained spread over our problem up to the present time.

Descartes (1596–1650) was the first who posed questions about the solar system in the modern sense. In order to understand his theory, let us imagine ourselves to be the spectators when street-sweepers have thrown a cartload of dust from a bridge into an eddying river. What does one see when looking at the river from the bridge? In the centre of every eddy matter will collect and rotate. The heaviest dust-ball in the largest eddy represents the Sun. In the largest eddy smaller eddies move round the centre. The dust-balls concentrated in the smaller eddies are the planets. Dispersed particles in the smaller eddies are the satellites which turn round the planets.

The facts reminding Descartes of primary and secondary eddies when considering the solar system were, of course, the coincidence of the orbital planes of the planets, the fact that the planets all move in nearly circular orbits in the same direction, and the fact that particles circulate more quickly the shorter their distance from the centre of every eddy. In the satellite systems these principles are repeated.

Christiaan Huygens (1629–1695), the famous Dutch physicist, criticized the Cartesian vortices. For instance, the required "direct" sense of rotation of the planetary vortices is in conflict with the decrease of the angular velocity with increasing distance from the centre in the solar vortex. We should, however, not forget that Descartes died before Newton (1642–1729) revealed the existence of general gravitation, that basic phenomenon the knowledge of which clarifies so much.

Descartes's interpretation of the planetary system as a set of material globes dragged along by one large eddy and by a number of smaller eddies in a turbulent medium filling the universe, remains ingenious. Deadly to the theory of Descartes were, of course, the comets, apparently not caring anything about the existence of that medium in which the whole solar system was wrapped. However, what does not exist *now* may have existed in the past, and the Cartesian vortices, apparently vanquished, have regained their places brilliantly in quite recent forms of the "nebular hypothesis".

Kant (1724–1802), the great German philosopher, considering the many nebulae in the universe discovered by contemporary astronomers, in particular F. W. Herschel (1738–1822), was the first to assume that the Sun is a condensation product of one of these nebulae. The Sun remained for a long time surrounded by the shapeless remnant of the cloud. This cloud rotated round the Sun. Kant was apparently wrong when trying to interpret the origin of this rotation, but this makes no difference to the result, which he conceived correctly. A nebula rotating round the Sun will flatten out and extend in one plane. A rotating nebulous disk of this kind functions extremely well as the archetype of the planetary system. The extension of the nebula in one plane and the revolution of all parts of it round the Sun in one and the same direction, are explained. The remaining problem is: How does the disk condense into separate globes? It was Kant's opinion that a tendency to such concentrations existed. Nuclei, formed locally, collected

12 The Origin of the Solar System

all the matter. The nebula resolved finally into a number of planets.

Now, before going into our discussion, we should derive arguments from "tidal forces".

6. Tidal Forces

THE essence and effect of the tidal interactions between any two celestial bodies are clarified most easily by the Earth–Moon system. The Moon is subjected to specific forces because it circulates round the Earth in such a way that one and the same hemisphere always faces the Earth (Fig. 3).

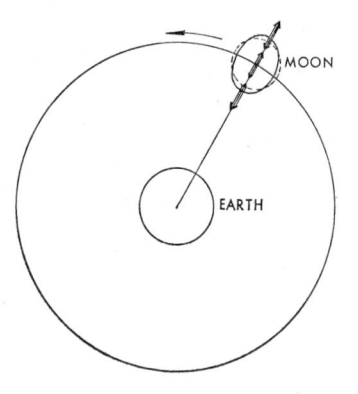

FIG. 3. Tidal forces of the Earth stretch the Moon out.

At the centre of the Moon, the Earth's attraction and the centrifugal force due to the Moon's motion in a circular orbit, are equal. An element of the Moon nearer to the Earth experiences stronger attraction and weaker centrifugal force, an element of the Moon further away from the Earth a weaker attraction and a stronger centrifugal force. Hence, the forces acting on the Moon result in a stretching of the moon-body in the direction of the Earth and in the direction away from it. These deformations are called "tidal deformations", and the forces causing them, "tidal forces".

The Moon is kept together by the gravitational attraction between its particles, and, at least when fluid, is deformed in such a way that the resultant of all forces acting at a point of its surface is perpendicular to this surface. The Moon's shape was proved to be an ellipsoid with the longest of its three axes directed toward the Earth.

Suppose, finally, that the Moon's volume would remain constant while its density would decrease. Then the Moon would be increasingly stretched. As soon as the tidal forces get stronger than the mutual attractions between the Moon's particles the Moon is destroyed. The Moon would suffer a similar fate if its constitution remained the same but its distance from the Earth decreased. This latter possibility will be touched on later. Here we note that a satellite can only exist when its density exceeds a certain critical value.

7. Does the Primeval Nebula Suffer Local Condensation?

LET us consider, within the Kantian disk, a certain small global element (Fig. 4) and ask the question whether this element will condense further. It was Roche who gave the answer, based on the knowledge we have just gained. The condensation will proceed when the density of the disk in that particular element exceeds a certain limit, depending on its distance from the Sun. The further away from the Sun the lower the threshold value of the density allowing conglomeration.

As a matter of fact, only in cases of rather high density do conditions occur in the Kantian disk such that planets are born.

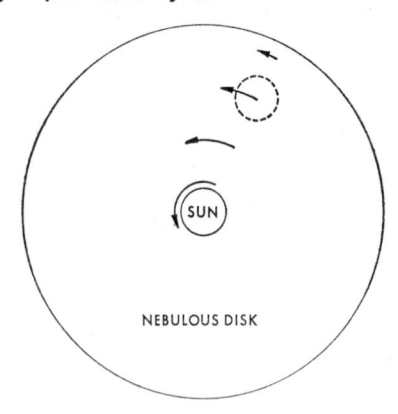

Fig. 4. Condensation of a given part of the primitive solar nebula against its dispersion by solar tidal forces is possible only when that part is sufficiently dense.

It is not difficult to prove, which Kant in his time did not realize, that when all the matter condensed in the planets today was dispersed and filled the primeval disk, extending beyond Pluto and showing a thickness of, say, the one-hundredth part of its diameter, the matter would have been much too rarified to show the slightest tendency towards agglomeration into planets.

Before discussing what circumstances might nevertheless have led to the result we are looking for, it is useful to review other theories.

8. Laplace's Theory

THE famous French mathematician Laplace (1749–1827), reformed the "nebular hypothesis".

A spinning gas cloud was thought to have extended beyond Uranus, the most peripheral planet known at the time. This cloud was subject to shrinking by cooling. This shrinking would be associated with an acceleration of the rotation of the cloud.

Laplace's Theory 15

Let us imagine the primitive nebula to be an only slightly flattened globe. The quicker the nebula's rotation the stronger its flattening. It will assume the typical form of a lens with a sharp edge. In fact, a moment will arrive when along its rim the centrifugal force balances gravitation. Consequently, if the nebula shrinks further, a ring of matter will liberate itself and not share in the further shrinking of the main mass (Fig. 5).

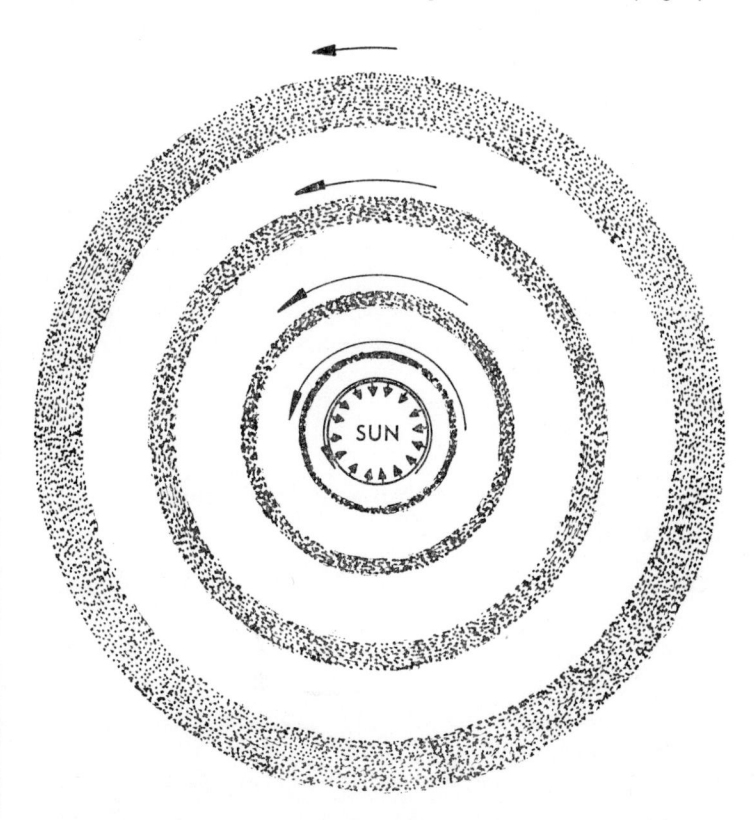

FIG. 5. Origin of the planetary system according to Laplace's hypothesis. The Sun, while contracting, releases again and again a gas ring along its equator.

Now, Laplace makes an additional assumption. The evolution should proceed in steps. Discontinuities in hydrodynamic processes are not as improbable as they may seem. A first ring is released, the nebula shrinks further and its rotation grows faster; a second ring is released and so on, the central portion of the nebula condensing to become the Sun.

9. Concentric Rings

WE MEET here without any doubt a very promising concept of the manner in which an extensive gas- or dust-cloud may change into a set of concentric rings, lying in one plane and turning round the Sun with velocities equal to those of the planets, while they move in circular orbits of the same average radius. Moreover, an evolution of this kind may explain why the radii of the rings are in a regular sequence, and hence, when the planets are formed, why their distances from the Sun are also in such a sequence.

10. The Position of the Axes of Rotation of the Planets

THE theory of Laplace seems to lead us so far that we really need to discuss some further details before considering the objections made against it. When analysing the possible structure of a gas ring turning round the Sun, we can easily state that this structure will not be stable. The ring will break up in knots pursuing each other in nearly one and the same orbit. As the times of revolution of these "cumuli" will never be exactly equal, they will overtake each other and finally assemble into one cloud.

This cloud, which is to change into a planet eventually

Position of the Axes of Rotation of the Planets 17

equipped with a satellite system, we shall call a "protoplanet". The last and second last remnants of a ring (Fig. 6) approach each other with an initially very low speed, from a relatively large distance. The bodies will attract each other with growing force as they come closer together. Consequently, the leading body will be decelerated, the following body accelerated. The leading body will start moving with a velocity lower than the

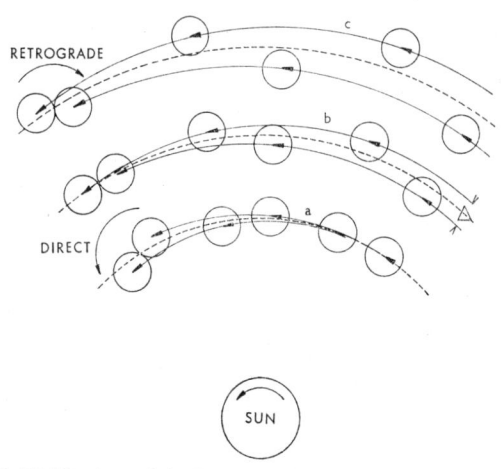

Fig. 6. Unification of the last two pieces of a ring will result in a protoplanet rotating in the direct sense (a), however, in limiting cases of original orbital radii differing more than Δ (b) in a protoplanet rotating in the retrograde sense (c).

Kepler velocity, the following body with a velocity higher than the Kepler velocity. Thus the leading body will be pulled in a little, the pursuing body pushed out a little. When they meet and unite this will always result in a tendency of the protoplanet to rotate round an axis perpendicular to the plane of its orbit and in a direction similar to the direction of revolution.

Moreover, a closer view, offered by Halm, reveals a characteristic difference Δ between the radii of the original orbits of the two uniting bodies, so that, if the actual difference is smaller than Δ the protoplanet will rotate in the "direct" sense, whereas, if the actual difference is greater than Δ the protoplanet will rotate in the reverse sense. Consequently, our surprise at discovering peripheral "retrograde" satellites in some systems is certainly not as justified as it seemed to be.

11. Gas Rings Round a Star Possible

ALL this gave H. Poincaré (1854–1912), the great French mathematician, reasons to support fully Laplace's cosmogony and to improve it in many ways. For instance, Poincaré showed that a gaseous ring turning round the Sun can really exist. Jeans (1877–1946) had pointed out that such a ring, if moving with the same angular velocity throughout, that is, like a rigid body, cannot be stable, but must expand. He neglected, however, the possibility that the ring moves with an angular velocity that decreases with increasing distance from the centre. If gas rings of this kind are possible structures, they may also form and disintegrate at a later stage, the pieces finally assembling into protoplanets.

O. Struve became convinced of the actual existence of gas rings round some close double stars. He ventured even to suppose that the formation of gas rings round such pairs is a rather frequent occurrence. On the other hand, Saturn's rings, although granular, are not much different from gas rings, if this gas is assumed to consist of very heavy molecules.

12. The Trojans

STILL another remarkable aspect of the planetary system proves indirectly the plausibility of initial planetary rings. When a planet moves round the Sun in a circular orbit, any free particle moving in the same circular orbit will eventually be united with the planet. The particle nearly always has a position relative to the planet which it will leave in course of time and never occupy again. There are, however, two positions which Lagrange (1736–1813) proved to be singular (Fig. 7). When a particle circulates at a distance from the planet, such that the planet, the particle, and the Sun occupy the corners of an equilateral triangle, the position is "stable". If the particle is

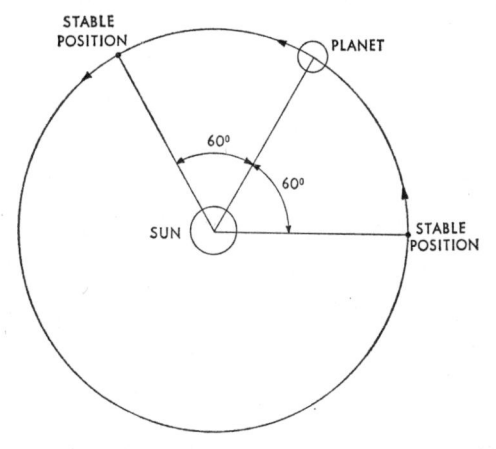

FIG. 7. The two stable positions of an asteroid with respect to a planet pointed out by Lagrange. The Trojans occupy these positions with respect to Jupiter.

forced to move away from this position by some slight perturbation, it will return after some time, perhaps overshoot the mark, but return again. The natural play of forces thus makes the particle oscillate about this particular position.

Now, these cases are realized. A small group of asteroids—Achilles, Patroclus, Hector, Nestor, Priamus, and Agamemnon (the Trojans)—occupy the first, others the second stable position. They confirm the correctness of Lagrange's theory. The small perturbations do not disturb the relative positions of the Trojans. They stay in these stable positions. The question arises: Do not the Trojans contribute a great deal to the proof that Jupiter is a condensation product of a primitive ring? The few remnants of the ring which were near Lagrange's "equilateral" positions towards the end of the condensation process have remained there ever since.

13. The Flat Disk Archetype

POINCARÉ gave the proof of a theorem which Kant anticipated. Non-elastic collisions of its particles will oblige a spinning gas- or dust-cloud to assume the shape of a flat disk. This is an important result. A gaseous solar cloud will not do this, because its molecules are perfectly elastic, but one consisting of dust particles will always degenerate into a pancake structure.

With this thesis, however, we are deviating from the promising ring idea supported by Laplace, and it must be conceded that it is very difficult to follow this idea further. In fact "heavy gunnery against Laplace's fortification" was fired on the basis of the following argument.

The contraction of the solar nebula having proceeded, ring after ring having been released, each predestined to become a planet, and the Sun having ended as the strongly concentrated mass exceeding the total mass of the planets by 740 times, what should have been the Sun's rate of rotation?

The solar rotational period is about one month. This period may seem reasonable, but in fact Laplace failed to make comprehensible why the Sun does not rotate in a few hours only. The argument is that after having shed its last ring, that which generated Mercury, the Sun must have shrunk further to its present radius, which is not greater than one-eightieth of the radius of Mercury's orbit. Why should solar rotation not have been speeded up accordingly?

14. The Dualistic Conception of the Solar System

THE puzzling slowness of the Sun's rotation brought forward an old idea. Buffon (1707–88) had already expressed the opinion that the Sun might have been hit by a comet. Due to this collision, pieces of matter would have been pushed out of the solar body. These pieces, rotating and turning round the Sun, would have survived as planets.

In Buffon's days the masses of comets, and the effect of collisions of comets with the planets or with the Sun, were often greatly overestimated, but this does not affect the principle which has reappeared in every modern "dualistic conception" of the planetary system.

Arrhenius (1859–1927) was the first to suggest a collision of the Sun with a foreign star. This collision resulted in the ejection of matter from both stars. Part of this matter continued to move round the Sun, forming a gaseous disk into which solid nuclei penetrated from outside. The planets condensed on the nuclei (Fig. 8).

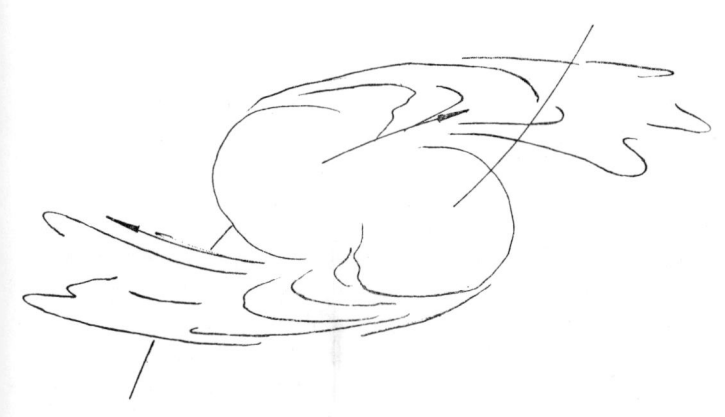

FIG. 8. Sketch of the events when two stars collide.

The foreign star must have departed, because when two stars coalesce, the ejected matter can only disappear into space or drop back on the resultant central body. Only the independence of two bodies A and B after the collision, opens the possibility that the matter expelled by A is directed by B into elliptic orbits round A.

Now, in order to achieve this result no direct collision between the Sun and a foreign star is required. Jeffreys pointed out that a direct collision would explain more easily why the protoplanets started to rotate in the direction of their revolution. However, if this argument is not accepted, the "tidal theory" is the most promising alternative.

15. The Tidal Theory in its Original Form

MOULTON and Chamberlin were the first to discuss the possible consequences of a close meeting of the Sun and a foreign star. An event of this kind must be counted among the possibilities.

Stars are assembled in clusters and island universes, spiral nebulae—immense whirls in space like our galaxy. The Sun and other stars in its neighbourhood make, as was pointed out by Oort, one revolution round the central axis of this great system in about 200 million years. Stars, however, while taking part in these general rotations, have their "proper motions" that might bring them close together at certain times. Of course it is impossible to indicate in the sky the particular star which passed near to the Sun and gave birth to the planetary system between 5000 and 10,000 million years ago, but we know how to depict what may have happened during such an encounter. A small body within short distance of a big one, for instance a satellite within short distance of a planet, must exceed a certain mass to avoid being robbed of its tidal bulges.

The Tidal Theory in its Original Form

If a foreign star heavier than the Sun came shooting past, then this foreign star may have torn matter away from the Sun. This matter would have formed two gaseous trails (Fig. 9). Due to the high velocity of the foreign star, both trails would have been curved. They would have started revolving

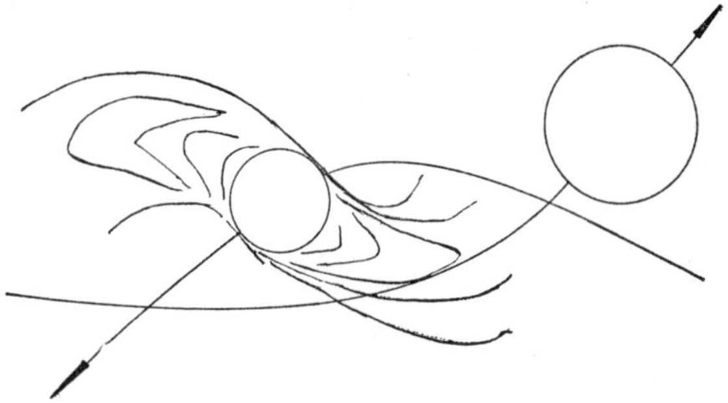

FIG. 9. Sketch of the events when two stars have a near meeting.

round the Sun as a spiral nebula. The more or less dense parts of it would have presented the first rude scheme of the planetary system. The gaseous trails in the opinion of Moulton and Chamberlin would cool down quickly. The gas would condense into solid particles revolving round the Sun—"planetesimals". The planets would be conglomerations of planetesimals.

It will appear later that Moulton and Chamberlin's "planetesimal-hypothesis" was basically correct. However, let us not try to explain the rule of Titius and Bode along the lines indicated here. We would never succeed.

16. The Tidal Theory in its Final Form

JEANS gave the tidal theory a new and more efficient form. He emphasized that the tidal force of the foreign star at the point of the Sun nearest to that star was slightly stronger than

24 The Origin of the Solar System

the force at the counterpoint (Fig. 10). Consequently, matter is torn away from the Sun mainly from one side. The Sun gets a tail which moves after the foreign star. After the departure of the foreign star no more gas will be torn away from the Sun. On the other hand, not all the gas will have followed the star. A kind of curved cigar is liberated. This cigar will not remain as one continuous mass. It will be split up into knots.

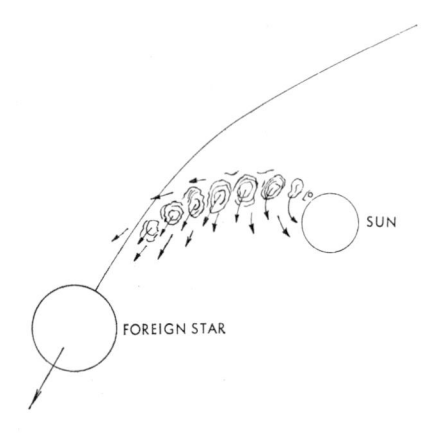

Fig. 10. Sketch of the creation of the planetary system according to Jeans's tidal theory.

However, the matter, when leaving the Sun, must have been very hot. Why should it not expand further? Only if this expansion were counteracted by strong forces could knots form and be concentrated into planets. Each of them would possibly have continued to move round the Sun. The orbital planes of these protoplanets may also have nearly coincided.

One more aspect suggests this solution. After the departure of the foreign star, part of the matter torn from the Sun will fall back on it. The effect of this fall may well be compared with the effect of the fall on the Sun of matter having circulated inside the orbit of Mercury. If this occurs the Sun will assume a rotation in the same direction as the revolution of the planets. As a matter of fact the Sun *is* rotating in the "direct" sense.

Woolfson brought forward arguments in favour of the opposite possibility. The materials forming the solar nebula were captured by the Sun from a light diffuse star passing close by. An encounter of this kind may indeed have been more efficient than any other encounter.

17. The Gain Obtained by Tidal Interaction

THE tidal hypothesis was favoured rather more than the theory of Laplace because a foreign star could have provided the planets with their high orbital velocities, whereas the speed of rotation of the Sun could be derived from a small rest mass dropping down on to it. The puzzling slowness of the solar rotation was thus easily explained. The way towards a dualistic conception of the planetary system seemed clear.

Some teaser once said that Jeans "bombed a camp of quietly deliberating astronomers" with his foreign star. Certainly the tidal theory had an extremely persuasive influence. Most students of our problem received the impression that there was no way out of the difficulties without the aid of a foreign star.

Computations were made of the number of times a foreign star will approach the Sun to within a distance from the Sun of, say, the distance of the planet Neptune. The age of the Earth, about 5000 million years, fixes the time when the foreign star gave birth to the planetary system as between 5000 and 10,000 million years ago.

The present wide dispersion of stars, even within the Milky Way, would on this reckoning have allowed only one star out of millions to raise a family of planets.

18. Is the Planetary System Unique?

IF WE were obliged to assume that our planetary system is a phenomenon of such extreme rarity, should we be surprised? Let us be honest and say yes. However, why should this planetary system not be unique? Why should the Earth not be the only globe in the universe lodging living creatures? Is the Creator not equally lavish with millions of spermatozoids, when only one, quite randomly, gets the chance to fertilize an egg-cell?

Yet part of the initial surprise would still remain if twentieth-century discoveries had not affected its foundations. The chance of a close encounter between the Sun and a foreign body in that far past in which it apparently happened, between 5000 and 10,000 million years ago, was many times greater than at present.

19. The Expanding Universe

LEMAÎTRE was the first to draw a remarkable conclusion from general relativity. The Universe cannot be in a stable state; it must be expanding. Eddington immediately gave full support to this hypothesis. Several investigators have discussed the possibility that reality is deceiving us, or that the Universe which is now expanding will not run out into emptiness, but will contract again in the future. Although modern natural philosophy rejects Nietzsche's conception of the "ewige wiederkehr des gleichen", it is suggested that the Universe is pulsating. This would deliver us from the alarming impression that the Universe should have been conceived at zero hour in an extremely dense condition and have been expanding ever since.

Now, something happened that, in problems of this magnitude, is very rare. The observations made by Hubble and his associates confirmed Lemaître's theory in an outstanding manner. The "snapshot" of the Universe made in our time is covered in all aspects by modern physics. It reveals an expansion of the Universe comparable with the inflation of a balloon. If small marks are made on an expanding balloon, we observe a gradual increase in the mutual distances between the marks. Moreover, the greater these mutual distances the greater the speed with which they move away from each other.

The small marks on our balloon are an analogue of the immense spiral nebulae, whose positions in the Universe are millions of light years apart. Indeed, all spiral nebulae move away from our home, the galaxy, with velocities proportional to distance. Looking backward from the present revelation of the Universe to what happened roughly 10,000 million years ago, we state a higher concentration of matter in a smaller space.

Did the Universe explode like a nuclear bomb? Only one conclusion is important here. All cosmic masses in any form, as gas clouds or as condensed stars may have interacted more strongly between 10,000 and 5000 million years ago than they get the chance to do at the present time. A dualistic conception of the solar system is reasonable.

20. Was it a Catastrophe at the Start?

NEITHER strong tidal interaction during a very short interval nor a collision between two stars can ever have resulted, even in rough outline to the planetary system as we know it now. According to Jeans and Jeffreys the solar gas-trail was condensed directly into planets and systems of satellites. The satellite systems would, in this case, have been created out of secondary gas-trails ejected by each of the protoplanets at the time when they made their first perihelion passage, as it is then that they are subjected most strongly to solar tidal forces.

However, whether trails of this kind will ever condense, rather than expand, is a matter for serious doubt. But even if protoplanets are directly formed, we can hardly think of their motions other than in highly eccentric orbits round the Sun. How could these orbits have become almost circular? Jeans and Jeffreys could answer this question only by stressing the resistance that the condensing planets would experience in the non-condensed remnants of the cloud. Hence we must consider first the possibility of a "resisting medium" taking part in the evolution of the solar system.

21. Did a Resisting Medium Do the Job?

THE influence of resisting media of different constitution and proper motion on the course of a planet has been investigated in detail by Nölke. He was able to prove that a medium dispersed through the solar system cannot have changed the eccentricities of the planetary orbits to any significant extent, unless it formed a solar nebula of a mass amounting to a large multiple of the total mass of the planets. Whether the planets, during their motion in eccentric orbits, assemble parts of the resisting medium or not, is of minor importance only. In any case the interaction between planets and medium must have been such as to change the orbits of the planets from markedly elliptic to nearly circular ones.

This conclusion was strong enough to lead to a complete revision of the tidal theory as formulated in the early works of Jeans and Jeffreys. How, for instance, could planets have acquired satellites? A much better picture of the evolution of the planetary system is the following.

More than 98 per cent of the matter leaving the Sun consisted of hydrogen and helium. These gases started to circulate round the Sun as an extensive cloud. Moving through this cloud are the protoplanets—conglomerations of meteorites consisting of the cooling and crystallizing substances of much rarer occurrence. The big planets, those who could bear their own atmosphere of hydrogen and helium, gathered from the cloud a large part of their mass. The smaller planets experienced only a reduction in the eccentricities of their orbits.

What remained of the hydrogen and helium atmosphere must, as was pointed out by von Weizsäcker, have been slowly dissipated. This may explain why we do not observe today any remnants of the initial solar nebula. However, a serious objection still remains. Is it possible that the foreign star could transfer sufficient orbital velocity to the matter extracted from the Sun in the event of the foreign star hitting or nearly hitting the Sun? The answer is decidedly negative unless the Sun at the meeting was a rarified giant star. This possibility, however, can hardly be accepted because, as far as we know, at the time of the creation of planets, 5000 million years ago, the Sun was well on the way to its present state.

As a consequence of these objections, two other dualistic theories have come to take the place of the tidal theory.

22. The Theories of Lyttleton and Hoyle

LYTTLETON assumed that the Sun in an early stage was one of the components of a double star. The other component was hit by a third star and expelled from the system, while our Sun became enveloped by a cloud which condensed finally into planets (Fig. 11). Later, Lyttleton developed the idea that the Sun once had two companions which collided and left the scene.

Hoyle also assumed the initial existence of a double star, one

30 The Origin of the Solar System

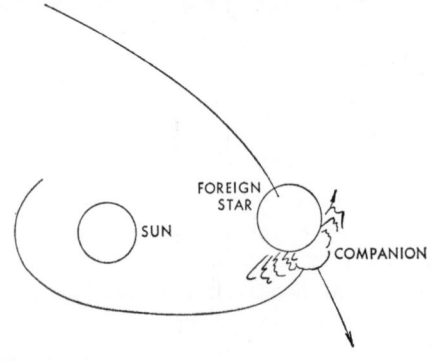

FIG. 11. Sketch of the creation of the planetary system according to Lyttleton's hypothesis. A companion of the Sun is hit by a foreign star.

of whose components exploded with great violence, that is became a "supernova". Almost the whole star, consisting mainly of hydrogen and helium was flung out into space. A small part of the star, mostly matter of higher molecular weight, was captured by the Sun, the unexploded component of the double star. In this way the Sun became surrounded by a gas or dust disk out of which the planetary system was formed (Fig. 12).

We should consider one particular aspect of these new forms of the dualistic conception of the planetary system. They settle a puzzling question.

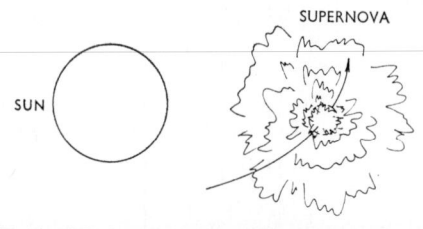

FIG. 12. Sketch of the creation of the planetary system according to Hoyle's hypothesis. A companion of the Sun explodes.

Almost beyond doubt the atoms of all kinds are built up in sequence of weight, from the elementary hydrogen at least up to iron in the interior of the stars. The still heavier elements, up to the radioactive ones, such as uranium and thorium, are probably formed during stellar explosions. After having left the stars that have synthesized them, these radioactive substances decay and show a certain "age". Now, since several of these substances were found in the Earth's crust and their age determined, we are informed about the time when the Earth condensed. As the date when this occurred 4700 million years ago is mostly given. Moreover, we may estimate how long the solar nebula existed before the planets were born. The conclusion seems to be that a star has been destroyed and has delivered the cloud of materials requested to form the planetary system, a rather short time only before this formation started.

An extremely rare event? Perhaps not. Although very old stars exist, reaching ages up to 10,000 million years (stars generated shortly after the birth of the entire universe) the contraction of the Sun and equally so of other near members of a star cluster, ready to cooperate, did apparently occur not earlier than 5000 million years ago. In an early cluster stage collisions between stars may have been rather frequent. On the other hand, stars in quite normal evolution seem to pass at some critical date through the explosive stage at which they become a "supernova". Hence, a solar companion of large mass may well have reached that instable state a long time ago, whereas the Sun, almost certainly will remain quiet for a long time to come.

23. The Hypothesis of Dauvillier

DAUVILLIER is of the opinion that a solution on the tidal basis lies in the complete dualism characterizing all events. He seriously considers, as opposed to Jeans, both of the spiral arms extracted from the Sun by the foreign star (Fig. 13).

32 The Origin of the Solar System

Assuming that both gas-trails deliver planets at their current distances, all of them are born as twins. Each pair of twins moved, originally separate, in two strongly eccentric orbits round the Sun. The two orbits, however, are mirrored with respect to the centre. Hence the twins must collide one day. They fuse together into one protoplanet, moving in an almost circular orbit round the Sun. Secondaries were formed in the same manner as their primaries once were.

This hypothesis, with its emphasis on unrealistic symmetries, might have been left out of account had not a new aspect, the influence of electric forces, been mentioned.

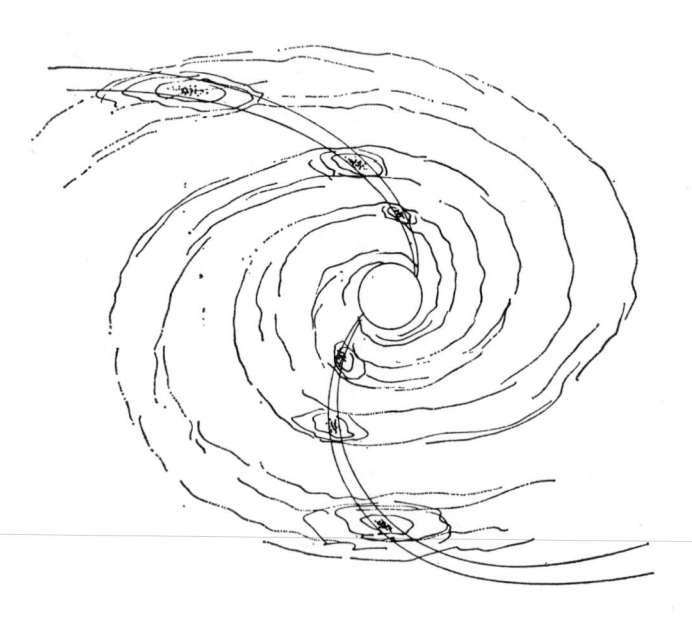

FIG. 13. Sketch of the creation of the planetary system according to Dauvillier's hypothesis. Each planet originated two-fold.

24. Did Electric Forces Enter the Scene?

DAUVILLIER took into account not only the two spiralling gas trails, but also the condensing influence of the two "jet streams" of electrons ejected by the Sun in the same two directions but only very slightly curved (Fig. 13).

Birkeland had already made a study of the orientating influence that the solar magnetic field might have executed during the development of the planetary system. Birkeland even saw a set of concentric rings originate from the streams of ions which leave the Sun continuously and are curved by the solar magnetic field towards concentric circles. The smaller the ratio between charge and mass of the ion, the greater the circle on to which it converges (Fig. 14).

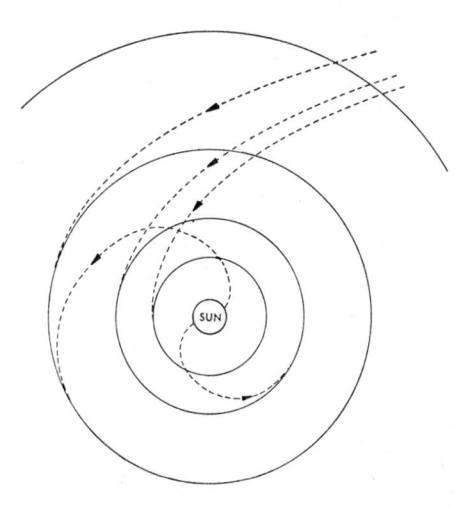

FIG. 14. Summary of the possible deflections of ion motions in the electromagnetic field of force of the Sun, pointed out by Birkeland and Alfvén.

Alfvén opened the door to the play of electromagnetic forces in cosmogony wider than did Birkeland, and in general with good reasons. These forces had been underestimated relative to general gravitation for a long time. Turbulent cosmic clouds are subjected strongly to these forces.

Now, among these cosmic clouds, we meet the early solar nebula, still consisting for the greater part of gaseous hydrogen and helium. Consequently, according to Alfvén, and supported by Lüst and Schlüter, electromagnetic interactions with the ionized primeval solar nebula may have been braking the rotation of the Sun's magnetic body to its present puzzling slowness. This process was almost certainly stimulated by the intervention of the Sun's own "corpuscular" rays.

It is, however, very doubtful whether solar magnetism has ever been strong enough to play the part Birkeland and Alfvén assigned to it in the further evolution of the planetary system. The author, too, must confess to have adhered in his first studies to similar assumptions, although taking into account electrostatic forces only.

Since it had become obvious that the theory of Laplace had to be discarded, it seemed almost naïve to look for the necessary governing principle in pure mechanics. Yet, at present, no student of our subject would dare to assume that electromagnetism has opened to us a clear way through the problems of the genesis of planets and satellites.

25. A Good Start Is Half the Work (Dutch Proverb)

THE origin of the planetary system, in the narrower sense of its conception, depends on the wrapping of the Sun in a gas- or dust-cloud. With the creation of a solar nebula the evolution of the planetary system is only just starting, and hence we are still confronted with the vital question of what mechanism dominated the evolution of the planetary system from this point on.

26. The Internal Friction of the Gas

THE force we have to take into account from this point on is "internal friction". It finds its expression in "viscosity". How does viscosity act and what does it contribute towards the changes of shape and motion of the primeval solar cloud?

Friction appears wherever material particles in close contact move with different velocities. In such cases kinetic energy is transferred from the one particle to the other. This process causes "dissipation" of energy. The complicating fact, however, is that a fraction of the total energy of any piece of matter exists as kinetic energy of its molecules, that is as heat. Hence, viscosity causes also transfer of heat, although part of this transfer is due to radiation. Now, notably the annihilation of temperature differences in a material body, be it gaseous, liquid, or solid, means loss of energy.

In short, viscosity is associated not only with dissipation of energy but also with loss of energy.

27. The Theorem of Minimum Loss of Energy due to Viscosity in Steady Motion

HELMHOLTZ, Korteweg, and Lord Rayleigh discovered a fundamental hydrodynamic principle that may be formulated as follows: a gaseous or liquid mass, whose parts are in relative motion, will seek conditions of motion associated with minimum loss of energy by viscosity.

36 *The Origin of the Solar System*

We can imagine this gaseous or liquid mass to rotate as a solid body. During a motion of this kind no energy is dissipated. Consequently, this will be the mode of motion any gaseous or liquid mass will try to assume. If this form of motion is attainable the gaseous or liquid mass will also assume a shape of revolution of some sort. The type fitting the motion, if the density is constant throughout the body, was proved by Newton to be a rotational ellipsoid. This is the shape, so well known, of the rapidly spinning planets, such as Jupiter and Saturn (Plates III and IV), but illustrated too, although in a less spectacular manner, by slower-spinning planets such as the Earth. Hence, every rotating gaseous or liquid mass will strive after uniform axial rotation, i.e. every part having the same angular velocity.

28. Steady Conditions Associated with Non-uniform Axial Rotation

IN VERY many practical cases the spinning mass will not succeed in assuming uniform axial rotation, simply because other factors intervene continuously.

Consider, for example, our Sun. Its equatorial period of rotation amounts to 25 days, whereas its polar period of rotation amounts to no less than 34 days. If the solar globe is supposed to be solid at a certain depth and to rotate with the polar period, equatorial west winds blow with a speed of 2400 km/hr. Evidently, even in a relatively dense star such as the Sun, there is no question of uniform angular velocity, and the problem is not only how these differences in angular velocity *can* be maintained, but also why these differences *must* be maintained.

Consider another example within our own environment, the terrestrial atmosphere. The insolation causes easterlies in low latitudes and westerlies in moderate latitudes. This planetary wind system does not stop on account of solar radiation being constantly transferred into the kinetic energy of air currents. This kinetic energy is retransformed into heat and this heat is reradiated into space. Meanwhile the general atmospheric circulation is maintained. It is solar radiation which continuously supplies the energy that is lost by friction. Our terrestrial atmosphere is simply compelled to deviate from uniform rotation.

The source of energy sustaining that puzzling mode of solar rotation rests in the interior of the Sun where energy is generated by "nuclear" processes. The giant planets Jupiter and Saturn show modes of rotation similar to the solar mode. Zonal speeds along the equator are greater than those in moderate and higher latitudes. Opinions have differed with regard to the source of energy maintaining the non-uniformity of the rotation of these planets. It may be from their own heat, or it may be from solar radiation. It seems more probable that their own heat is involved. Whereas Jupiter's distance from the Sun varies by about 10 per cent and thus the amount of solar radiation received by Jupiter by about 20 per cent, the intensity of its atmospheric circulation does not suffer any measurable variations.

Jupiter and Saturn must have relatively hot interiors, which explains why these planets present surface temperatures slightly higher than the temperatures at which solar radiation would maintain them in equilibrium conditions.

29. Tendencies in the Primeval Nebula

RETURNING now to the primitive Sun and the nebula moving around it, we are confronted with the fundamental question of what shape and what mode of rotation the nebula will assume.

A first idea is easily obtained with the aid of three simplifying assumptions:

(a) The mass of the primeval nebula was a small fraction only of the solar mass,
(b) the temperature of the gas was everywhere the same,
(c) the gas is throughout of the same chemical composition.

According to the first condition, solar attraction dominates the mutual attractions between parts of the nebula, the second and third conditions demand that the density of the gas is proportional to its pressure everywhere.

The viscosity has a flattening effect and the primeval cloud will be deformed to a more or less thin disk. The different parts of the disk will acquire velocities of revolution which, since the mass of the disk is negligibly small, will differ only slightly from the velocity of any particle moving freely in a circular orbit round the Sun—the Kepler velocity. The slight differences between the actual angular velocity of an element of the nebula and the Kepler velocity are, when conditions have become steady, due to radial pressure gradients.

Now, if uniform temperature and chemical composition are realized, the angular velocity of the gas depends on the distance from the central axis only. The nebula rotates cylinderwise. If this is true, internal friction acts as if gas cylinder is rubbing against gas cylinder, while their angular velocity decreases outwards. Consequently, kinetic energy is transformed continuously into heat, the surplus energy being dissipated.

Yet, although the heat generated by internal friction is always partly lost, and the gas disk by the breakdown of its energy is liable to continuous reformation, an almost steady state is reached. Gerasimović was the first to show that this state is associated with the following relation between the angular velocity ω and the distance r from the centre:

$$\omega = c_1 + c_2 r^{-2}. \tag{2}$$

In this relation c_1 and c_2 are arbitrary constants. Nevertheless, the relationship can never be strictly realized because, when all cylinders are spinning with near Kepler velocities, the squares of their periods of revolution are proportional to the third powers of their radii. Hence, in this case,

$$\omega^2 r^3 = \text{constant} \tag{3}$$

and the fundamental question remains: What manner of rotation does the disk assume?

30. Dispersion of the Primeval Nebula

ONE of the answers to this question has been given by von Weizsäcker and Lüst (Fig. 15). The inner gas cylinders are pushed slowly towards the central axis, whereas the outer

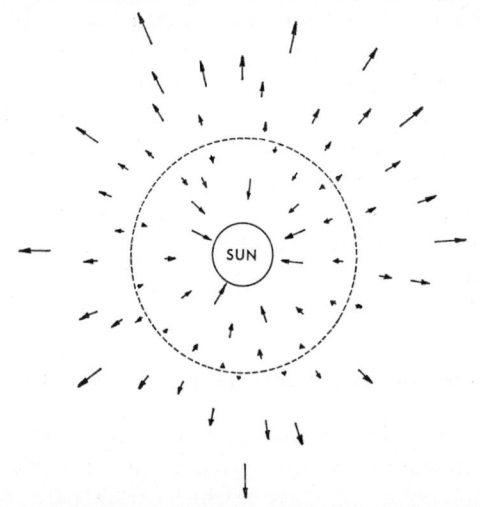

FIG. 15. Dispersion of the nebulous disk according to von Weizsäcker and Lüst. The part of the nebula inside a circular border contracts on the Sun, the part of the nebula outside the circular border expands into space.

ones are pushed slowly towards the periphery. Hence the disk will be dispersed partly by assimilation with the Sun, partly by radial dispersion in space.

The latter part of this process should not be taken too seriously. The development results in a slow expansion of the disk, the energy necessary for this expansion being supplied by the central region of the disk, while spiralling toward the Sun. An interesting detail is that the disk may temporarily become a ring.

The author was impressed by the fact that, whenever the gas disk, by gradual adjustment, approaches the ideal state of invariable structure, it does so along the lines of least resistance. Very probably the disk will not be divided in two belts only, a central one spiralling inward and a peripheral one spiralling outward, but into a set of belts, each divided into an inner zone moving towards the Sun and an outer zone moving away from the Sun. Along the fronts between these belts condensation of matter occurs in the zones between rarefaction. The gas disk will tend to be resolved into a set of concentric rings. This opens our view on the probability that nature itself bridges the gap between Kant's conception, the gas disk, and Laplace's conception, the set of concentric rings.

Before following this course with confidence, we must, however, consider other difficulties in cosmogony.

31. The Primeval Nebula—Was it Turbulent?

THE disk, so clearly revealing itself as the embryo of the planetary system, has been considered so far to be a quietly spinning mass of gas, a mass in which currents are "laminar", meaning that every layer moves smoothly over the adjacent one, in opposition to the wilder currents in a "turbulent" mass of gas (Fig. 16).

Now, laminar currents in any natural mass of gas may be disregarded. A laminar current can be produced experimentally between two plates, or in a tube, or wind tunnel, but the currents in our atmosphere, for instance, always involve larger or smaller eddies.

The difference between turbulent atmospheric currents and the experimental laminar currents is impressive. The internal friction in the first case is several thousands of times stronger

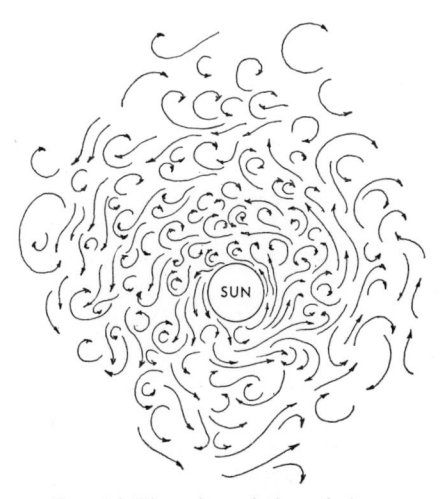

Fig. 16. The solar nebula turbulent.

than in the second case. The "viscosity" of the medium in turbulent motion depends on the behaviour of smaller and larger eddies. In laminar motions, however, viscosity depends on the behaviour of the molecules of the gas.

Structural variations in our terrestrial atmosphere would require a time interval several thousands of times as long if brought about by "molecular viscosity" than by the larger scale "eddy viscosity". Our knowledge of the terrestrial atmosphere is quite sufficient proof of the thesis that the viscosity in the primeval gas disk, which was to condense into planets, was also due to turbulence. If "molecular viscosity" had been the only agent, evolutionary changes which lasted, say, 1000 million years would have lasted millions of millions of years.

It is true that every extensive cloud in natural conditions is turbulent, but it is important to know what kind of turbulence is dominant. Aerodynamicists compare the smaller and larger eddies in a medium with the smaller and larger waves propagated through a medium, and use the term "turbulence spectrum" to characterize the prevailing conditions. Kolmogorov, Heisenberg, Chandrasekhar, and von Weizsäcker have studied these facts intensively.

The turbulence spectrum is observed almost directly in the plume of smoke from a factory chimney. A plume of this kind includes eddies of all sizes, but not equal numbers of all sizes. Among them are only a few very small ones. The number of eddies increases with increasing dimensions. After passing a maximum associated with a certain diameter, the number of eddies decreases with increasing dimensions. There are only a few very large ones.

The axes of these eddies are in general oriented in all directions. The eddies are constantly reformed and destroyed, reviving and killing each other. Randomness dominates this play of coming into existence and then perishing, but the spectral distribution of diameters is maintained.

Now, turbulence follows a fixed course within certain limits. Larger eddies are transformed into smaller eddies. Continuous degeneration takes place terminating in molecular viscosity. This raises the question as to how the greatest number of eddies can be of average dimensions, not of the smallest kind. The answer is that we must formulate steady conditions. Steady conditions mean that the largest eddies in the medium have to be created continuously. This happens in a pot of soup which is stirred. In fact the large eddies create smaller ones by "dissipation". This operation is associated with dissipation of energy. The dissipation is greater the smaller the eddies. The small eddies disappear, it is said, in the "dissipation pit".

If the spectrum of eddies is the same in all three directions, it is called "isotropic". An isotropic spectrum will occur only when there is no reason for different eddy magnitudes to occur in different directions. It is observed in those rarified nebulae floating in space in which the gravitational field has no specific direction, and in which the mutual attraction between parts is negligible.

Let us compare them with the eddy motions in our terrestrial atmosphere. The eddy motions in the plume of smoke leaving a chimney are approximately isotropic. They are of such small dimensions that gravitation is of no importance. Small-scale turbulence is as a rule isotropic. As soon as we consider large-scale turbulence the image changes.

Under what natural conditions do eddies occur? They occur in a gas or liquid when two currents move with different speeds along a boundary plane and when the relative speed of the currents exceeds a critical value, as was pointed out by Reynolds depending on the density of the gas or liquid. Then eddies originate whose axes coincide with the boundary plane.

Thus we meet eddies in a river near the pillars of a bridge, and eddies in the smoke plume of a factory chimney, caused by the wind blowing along the Earth's surface. Fixed walls act as brakes on the gas or liquid currents moving along them and this causes differences of speed that may result in a turbulent motion of the gas or the liquid.

Consider the winds at two different levels. The surface winds and the winds higher up differ; a vertical gradient of wind speed exists. The difference in wind speed causes the air to start rotating around horizontal axes. We have evidence of these eddies in the wavy rows of clouds which sometimes form. However, we know also that they remain small in comparison with cyclones about vertical axes. Why is this?

Every parcel of air moving upwards expands, every parcel of

air moving downward is compressed. The first parcel grows colder, the second parcel hotter. Hence, turbulence about horizontal axes costs more energy than turbulence about vertical axes. Thus when the gradient of wind speed coincides with the direction of gravitation, eddies will be created, but their dimensions will not be in the least comparable with the dimensions of the eddies which originate when the gradient of wind speed is directed horizontally, that is perpendicular to the direction of gravitation. Whereas the first eddies reach dimensions of the order of hundreds of metres, the others reach dimensions of the order of thousands of kilometres.

Now, it should be noted that in the gas or dust disk out of which the planetary system was created, the angular velocity decreased outwards. These differences of periods of revolution are a constant source of turbulence, and this turbulence breeds in the first place eddies of all dimensions, turning in a direction opposite to the direction of rotation of the whole nebula. The question is: To what extent does turbulence permit a certain regularity of rotation of the nebula, and to what extent is a certain order promoted?

Surveying the present system of planets moving in almost perfect circles in one and the same direction, in almost one and the same plane, the original turbulence can never have been violent. The primeval nebula must have become as flat as a pancake, and this structure is certainly not liable to isotropic turbulence if ever turbulence was important at all. The impression prevails that turbulence increased viscosity to such an extent that the main changes of structure of the original chaotic mass of gas occurred in short time on the cosmic scale, while turbulence and thus the viscosity of the gas decreased. In the pancake nebula small-scale turbulence must have been essentially reduced. Consequently, if much turbulence remained after the early formation of the solar nebula, vortices with axes perpendicular to its equatorial plane are the only type that can have remained.

The Primeval Nebula—Was it Turbulent? 45

With this in view, von Weizsäcker suggested that the initial disk has resolved itself into trails of persistent eddies (Fig. 17). Now, the formation of persistent eddies is a well-known phenomenon in experiments with streaming or rotating fluids. Even in our terrestrial atmosphere semi-permanent regions of low and high pressure exist where air moves round in a cyclonic or anticyclonic direction. The hypothesis that trails of vortices originated in the initial solar nebula gained importance because

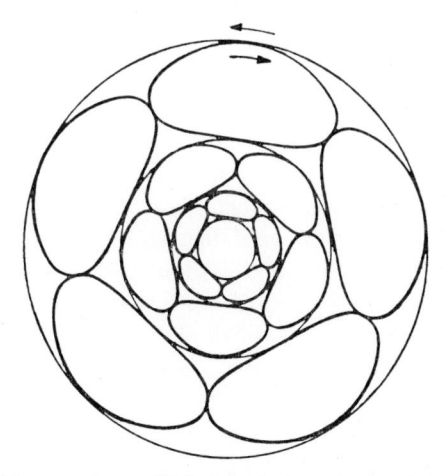

Fig. 17. Picture of von Weizsäcker's hypothesis of the natural resolution of the solar nebula in large vortices.

the pattern conceived by von Weizsäcker could be identified with the pattern of elliptic orbits of particles moving freely round the Sun, even orbits of considerable eccentricity. The structure of von Weizsäcker's nebula was apparently distinguished by a minimum frequency of collisions between the particles constituting it—a premise reminding us strongly of the principle of minimum loss of energy by viscosity. The urgently required principle creating order seemed to be revealed.

For this reason von Weizsäcker's hypothesis deserves an analysis in greater detail. Each trail of vortices is comparable with the circle of balls in a ball-bearing. This kind of motion must have caused the matter of the disk to condense in the ridges between which the vortices were circling round the Sun. Are the planets perhaps condensation products of these rings? We know how fruitful the conception of concentric rings has remained since Laplace.

However, von Weizsäcker's hypothesis was critized most strongly by the very investigators, Tuominen, Safronov, and others, who emphasized the inevitability of turbulence in the disk. In a few words: turbulence always signifies disorder. In von Weizsäcker's nebula, on the contrary, turbulence created order. Furthermore, why in such a turbulent mass of gas, should the molecules have been induced to move in certain orbits of least resistance, as if they were free? By their mutual collisions they actually never get the chance to behave in this way. Solar gravitation would have been directed perpendicular to the axes of these large vortices, a fact which, as was mentioned earlier, would have had a strong dissipating effect.

We need not be surprised therefore that Nölke and Jeffreys were able to show that von Weizsäcker's whirling cells, instead of being associated with minimum loss of energy, are in strong contradiction to this principle. These large vortices can never have spontaneously developed. They might have developed slowly in a quietly spinning primitive disk. The building up of trails of vortices in a disk that has already assumed a rather steady state of rotation *costs* energy.

For this reason many critics discarded von Weizsäcker's hypothesis immediately. Is this justified? Why should solar radiation not continuously contribute enough energy to sustain in the primitive nebula trails of mighty vortices, when similar trails are sustained in our terrestrial atmosphere, including "jet streams", round the world through both hemispheres in the higher airlayers? Do not the subtropical belts of high air-pressure prove to the meteorologist the natural existence of annular condensations in a rotating nebula where he did not expect them?

The author, therefore, was always ready to agree that von Weizsäcker's idea of a series of concentric gas- or dust-rings shows a certain parallelism with the way he indicated. However, the difficulties the satellite systems would have caused von Weizsäcker, if he had tried to explain them, would have been almost insurmountable.

32. Local Condensations Caused by Turbulence

THERE is one phenomenon associated with turbulence which Kuiper stressed in an attempt to explain how the condensation of the planets could have occurred directly from the gas disk. A serious objection against Kant's hypothesis was, as we know, that the gas disk would nowhere have sufficient density to allow the disk to clot. The tidal forces exercised by the Sun would prevent any condensation. The nebula would nowhere exhibit "gravitational instability", which means that the internal attraction of parts of the mass would be nowhere greater than the forces trying to pull them apart.

Kuiper suggested that variations of the density in a highly turbulent solar nebula and random transgressions above this density's threshold value might, in some places, have led to condensations such that further agglomerations into planets were stimulated. A further assumption, necessarily associated with this one, is that the total mass of the disk should have amounted to at least one-tenth of the solar mass. Otherwise the nebula would have nowhere shown sufficient density to become unstable and to bear planets. A requisite of Kuiper's hypothesis is that the initial masses of the planets must have been large multiples of their present masses.

33. The Different Chemical Composition of the Planets

THE planets are of very different structure (Table 6). Let us compare the extreme cases. Saturn has a mass exceeding the

TABLE 6. MASS AND RADIUS OF PLANET (EARTH = 1) AND MEAN DENSITY IN g/cm^3

Planet	Mass	Radius	Mean density
Mercury	0·054	0·38	5·46
Venus	0·814	0·96	5·06
Earth	1	1	5·52
Mars	0·107	0·52	4·12
Jupiter	317·5	10·97	1·33
Saturn	95·1	9·03	0·71
Uranus	14·5	3·72	1·55
Neptune	17·6	3·38	2·41
Pluto	0·05 ?	0·47 ?	2·9 ?

mass of the Earth 95 times. The average density of Saturn, however, is 0·7 only, whereas the average density of the Earth amounts to 5·5 g/cm^3.

In a heavier planet we expect stronger compression and higher density than in a lighter planet, provided their matter is of equal chemical composition. Now, Saturn matter may be in the gaseous state, Earth matter in the liquid or solid state. However, if this is the explanation for the difference of structure, Saturn temperatures should be so high as to disagree with the temperature actually measured at the planet's surface. Saturn's surface temperature is about 120°C absolute and thus higher, although not significantly higher, than the temperature which every globe would assume when placed at Saturn's distance from the Sun, if not heated from within.

As was mentioned earlier, Saturn probably possesses internal heating, but Saturn cannot glow in its interior and be relatively cool in its outer layers. In this case the planet would be brilliantly self-luminous. Such luminosity is not observed, and the only explanation of the large difference in density between Saturn and the Earth is that the latter is composed of relatively heavy and the former of relatively light substances.

The Earth has a liquid core with a radius of 3400 km, very probably consisting of iron and nickel, and perhaps a high pressure kind of silicates. The Earth bears a mantle of 2900 km thickness, consisting of well-known stony materials. Besides the iron in the core and some in the mantle, silicon, magnesium, and oxygen are the elements most frequently occurring on the Earth.

Kothari was the first to point out that Saturn cannot be built up out of these relatively heavy elements. Saturn must be built up out of relatively light elements, in particular carbon and nitrogen, while hydrogen and helium must contribute towards at least 69 per cent of its weight. Among the chemical combinations observed by spectroscopic methods in the atmosphere of Saturn, are high amounts of methane and ammonia. The oxygen, bound in water and carbonic acid, has probably moved toward Saturn's centre. The hydrogen and helium, although undoubtedly having moved towards Saturn's surface, are difficult to observe at the very low temperatures prevailing on this planet. The puzzling scarcity of hydrogen relative to helium in the atmospheres of Saturn and Jupiter is, according to Öpik, only comprehensible if hydrogen was frozen out. He ventures even to call Saturn and Jupiter "hydrogen snowballs".

Now, what do we know about the chemical composition of the planet's *a priori*? Is it certain that the matter condensing into planets, the matter composing the primeval nebula, was of the same chemical composition as solar matter?

34. The Primeval Nebula of Cosmic Composition

SOLAR matter can hardly differ much from average star matter. We note among the objects dispersed in the Universe, the large nebulae and individual stars, a chemical composition which is often designated as "cosmic composition". We give it in Table 7, borrowed from Russell and others, in the usual logarithmic form. To take one example, the weight of sodium and the weight of silicon in the cosmos are in the ratio of about 1:200.

TABLE 7. CHEMICAL COMPOSITION OF COSMICAL MATTER IN LOGARITHMIC SCALE (SILICON = 0)

Element	Logarithm	Element	Logarithm
Hydrogen	+4·54	Sulphur	−0·37
Helium	+3·68	Chlorine	−0·5
Carbon	+0·58	Argon	+0·3
Nitrogen	+0·88	Potassium	−2·18
Oxygen	+1·14	Calcium	−1·16
Fluorine	−1·0	Titanium	−2·58
Neon	+1·21	Chromium	−2·04
Sodium	−1·31	Manganese	−2·10
Magnesium	+0·03	Iron	−0·27
Aluminium	−0·06	Cobalt	−2·54
Silicon	0·00	Nickel	−1·42
Phosphorus	−1·8	Zinc	−2·56

Characteristic for cosmic composition is the presence of 86·5 per cent of the total weight of matter in the form of hydrogen and of about 12 per cent in the form of helium. The production of heat in all stars is due to the transformation of hydrogen into helium, the binding together of four hydrogen atoms into one helium atom—a process by which heat is liberated. Consequently the older stars must contain relatively more helium than the younger ones. What interests us here, however, is the almost necessary conclusion that the planets too are condensation products of matter consisting originally, for more than 98 per cent of hydrogen and helium.

Now, even Jupiter and Saturn contain a great deal less hydrogen and helium than cosmic matter. We have mentioned already the 69 per cent for Saturn. Similar computations made by Harrison Brown for the other big planets, lead to:

Jupiter	87	per cent
Saturn	69	per cent
Uranus	6	per cent
Neptune	0·5	per cent

Even if Jupiter was ever composed of cosmic matter its initial mass must have amounted to about ten times its present mass. Consequently Jupiter must have lost 90 per cent of its mass, *or* Jupiter has never been able to take possession of more than 10 per cent of the hydrogen and helium offered to it.

If the alternatives are posed this way, then, for instance, our own Earth should have lost at least 99 per cent of its original mass *or* should never have been able to accumulate the hydrogen and helium in any significant quantity.

35. When did the Primeval Nebula Lose its Hydrogen and Helium?

WHEREAS today the total mass of the planets is the 740th part of the solar mass, the mass of the primeval disk, according to Kuiper's estimate, should have amounted to the 10th part of the solar mass. Let us overlook here Ter Haar's doubt as to whether this proportion caused sufficient concentration of matter to overcome its dissipation due to the high degree of turbulence that has to be accepted. Instead, let us try to solve the problem of how the main part of the spinning matter, almost exclusively hydrogen and helium, was finally lost.

52 The Origin of the Solar System

One way was, as we know, pointed out by von Weizsäcker and Lüst. Part of the hydrogen and helium was to unite with the Sun, whereas an almost equal part was to withdraw into space.

This operation would have taken "only" 200 million years. Hence there is no difficulty from this side, and yet there is a snake in the grass. In fact, if the large mass of the initial disk had been real, even a small fraction of this mass united with the Sun would have provided it with the high rotational speed which the dualistic conception of the planetary system explained away so easily.

The electromagnetic coupling between the Sun and the massive primitive gas disk, no doubt ionized, might, as suggested by Alfvén, Lüst and Schlüter, have decelerated the solar spinning, but an almost greater difficulty is that the lost matter would have been active at first in accumulating planets and would have left the scene after this operation. Why should a planet first gather a large amount of matter by its own attraction and lose the greater part of it in a later stage? How could Jupiter lose the nine-tenth part of its mass, the Earth even the ninety-nine-hundredth part.

The Earth has no free hydrogen in its atmosphere, probably because this element is chemically active, but also no helium, the inert gas, although it is continuously delivered by natural sources. The light hydrogen and helium atoms fly about at remarkably high temperatures in the "exosphere" and consequently at such speeds that they leave our world whenever they get the chance. This simple fact makes it improbable that the Earth has ever possessed hydrogen and helium in any significant amount.

Kuiper has investigated whether the Sun by its "radiation pressure" might have blown substances, chiefly hydrogen and helium, away from the protoplanets. In that case hydrogen and helium might have been blown away from the central part of the primeval nebula—from the region where the terrestrial

When did the Primeval Nebula Lose its Hydrogen and Helium?

planets of high density originated. However, the Sun can hardly ever have had the capacity to do so. The intensity of the common solar radiation has probably increased and not decreased over the ages. The "corpuscular" solar rays or "solar wind", whose impacts and dragging force provide comets with particular kinds of tails, might, it is true, have stripped planets of the greater part of their mass, but this theory would meet almost equally strong objections as it involves the aprocryphal thesis that the planets have lost the greater part of their mass at a rather late stage.

The condensation of gas and dust to protoplanets would have been achieved in a relatively small interval after the evolution of the primeval nebula. Von Weizsäcker estimates the interval in which the density of the immense hydrogen and helium cloud decreased to half its value to be 5 million years. A transformation of this kind, however, must have reduced the turbulence in the nebula by a similar amount. Both factors reduce the probability of random assemblage of protoplanets very quickly. Hence, protoplanets would have formed in the early turbulent stage involving unstrained conditions, perhaps during 1 million years only. Kuiper even estimates spontaneous condensations by gravitation to have occurred between 10,000 and 100,000 years after the conception of the solar nebula. Consequently, the solar nebula must then have presented not only its greatest density, but also its highest degree of turbulence.

We should never forget that the planets themselves have developed satellite systems. Satellite systems must have been formed at an early date, and so the question arises whether these systems perhaps could have developed from the mother planet in its initial state.

Before answering this question it should be pointed out that when the mass of a planet decreases, the same is true of the attraction that keeps a satellite in its orbit. Hence this satellite must slowly move away from the centre. Processes of this kind may, of course, have occurred. We recognize a

54 The Origin of the Solar System

similar process in the recession of the Moon from the Earth. It is, however, certain that for such recession there was in many cases decidedly no room. If the mass of a planet decreases to one-tenth of its original mass a satellite will withdraw in the same time-interval to 10 times its original distance from the centre. Even in the case of Jupiter an effect of this magnitude would have had serious consequences. Its innermost satellite V circulates at a distance from the centre only slightly greater than five planet radii.

Now, what are we to think of Mars, whose inner satellite Phobos circulates at a distance from the centre not greater than three planet radii? This satellite's period of revolution is even shorter than the planet's period of rotation. The author has been unable to obtain any plausible picture of the origin of Mars and its two minuscule satellites from a protoplanet at least as big as Saturn. This giant planet would have developed a small terrestrial core and within its wrapping a pair of very much smaller "stones". It would have evaporated and been blown away by "solar wind" save for this core and the two little stones.

36. Temperatures in the Primeval Nebula

AFTER this detour, let us return to our starting point, that is the pattern of some inner terrestrial planets consisting of relatively heavy substances and some outer big planets consisting of relatively light substances.

One factor, not yet taken into account, is the temperature of the gas in the initial disk when giving birth to planets. Evidently this temperature cannot have deviated much from the temperature that is assumed by every small particle when absorbing solar radiation and emitting it again. Table 8 contains the temperatures of the gas near every planet in "radiative equilibrium" with the Sun.

TABLE 8. ABSOLUTE TEMPERATURE AT THE SURFACE OF A PLANET IN RADIATIVE EQUILIBRIUM WITH A SOLAR TEMPERATURE OF 5800° CELSIUS, ABSOLUTE, OR °KELVIN

Mercury	470°K
Venus	340
Earth	290
Mars	240
Asteroids	180
Jupiter	130
Saturn	90
Uranus	70
Neptune	50

TABLE 9. PHYSICAL CONSTANTS OF VARIOUS SUBSTANCES. TEMPERATURES IN °CELSIUS, ABSOLUTE, OR °KELVIN

Substance	Molecular weight	Melting point	Boiling point
Water	18	273°K	373°K
Carbon dioxide	44	195	217
Ammonia	17	195	240
Methane	16	89	112
Neon	20/22		27
Helium	4		4
Hydrogen	2		20

Table 9 shows the boiling point and the freezing point at normal atmospheric pressure of a number of the main constituents of the planets. Only those substances which are in the gaseous or liquid state within the region of the planetary system are included. The metals and inorganic compounds are not included. Silicon dioxide is certainly the most important of the substances which give the terrestrial planets their solidity.

Some readers will be surprised at the attention Table 9 pays to the inert gas, neon. However, in the cosmos this gas seems to occupy the third place after hydrogen and helium, as illustrated in Table 7.

37. Gases, Liquids, and Solids in the Primeval Nebula

W E LEARN from Tables 8 and 9 that hydrogen, helium, and neon exist as gases throughout the entire solar system. Only the giant planets, Jupiter and Saturn, managed to seize an important quantity of these elements.

When moving away from the Sun, we notice that water condenses near Venus and freezes between the Earth and Mars. Carbonic acid condenses near Mars and freezes in the belt of asteroids. Ammonia also crystallizes in this belt. Methane, however, does not solidify before we approach Saturn. It certainly is of the greatest importance that the transition from gas to liquid and solid is achieved for more than one planetary constituent near Mars and further outward. The curious swarm of asteroids certainly does not circulate by chance there where the planets change from small and heavy to large and light. The impression prevails that a planet in development between Mars and Jupiter grew too large for the smaller scale and too small for the larger scale and was destroyed.

Another important conclusion may be drawn. Planets grow only in an area where sufficient materials in the solid phase are available, or where substances showing at least a tendency to form small crystals, "ice germs", are available. In order to refine the notion of such germs it should be remembered that in our atmosphere, raindrops do not condense unless the "vapour pressure" is so high that an equal number of molecules per second plunge into the drop as evaporate from it. This limits the "maximum vapour pressure".

The maximum vapour pressure increases with temperature. It is, however, also largely dependent on the kind of water surface relative to which vapour pressure is measured. In order to make raindrops, small water globules floating in the air, a much higher vapour pressure or a much lower temperature is

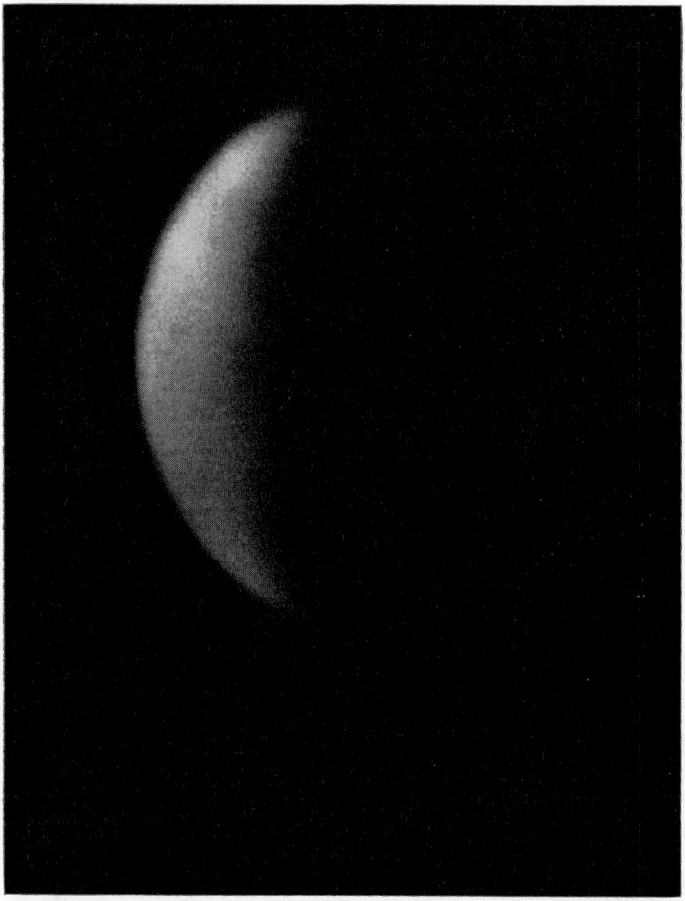

PLATE I. Most similar dense terrestrial neighbour, Venus, completely cloud-covered, showing almost no rotation. (*Reproduction permission Pic du Midi.*)

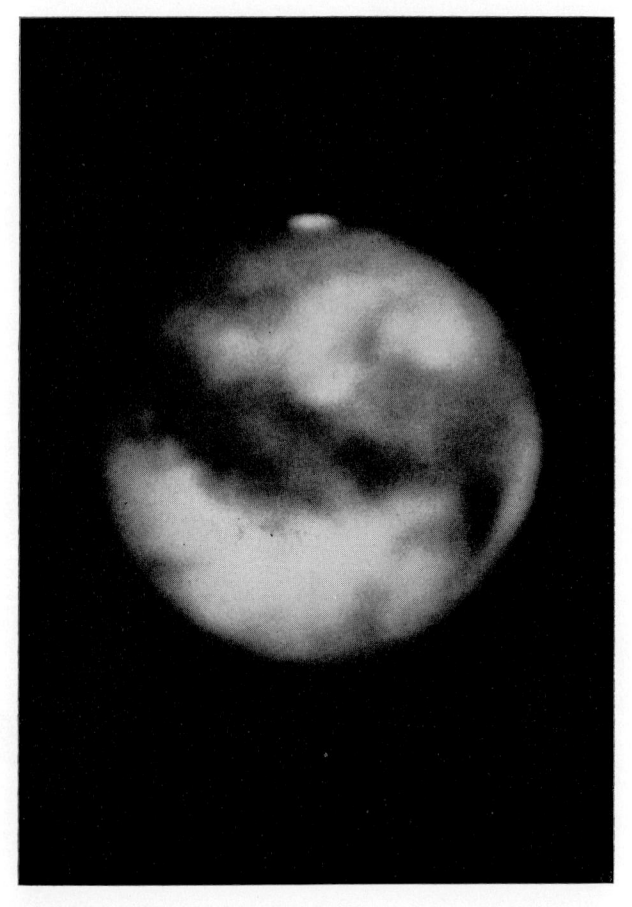

PLATE II. Well-known small terrestrial neighbour, Mars. Clear surface markings, clouds observed incidentally, one snow-covered pole in winter season. (*Reproduction permission Pic du Midi.*)

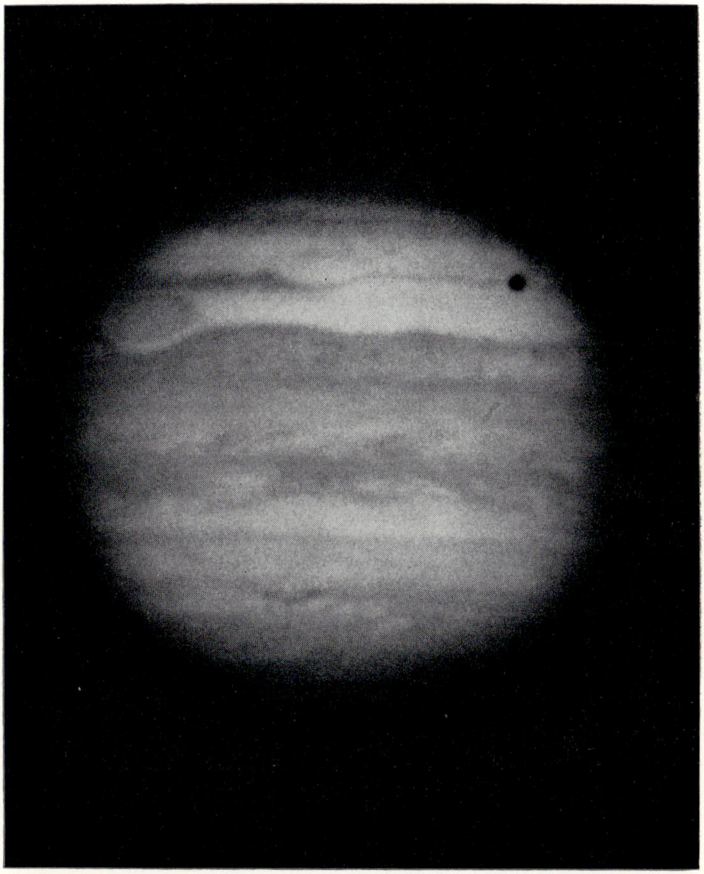

PLATE III. Major planet Jupiter, rotating quickly, with famous red spot in its clouds, during satellite Europe's crossing. (*Reproduction permission Pic du Midi.*)

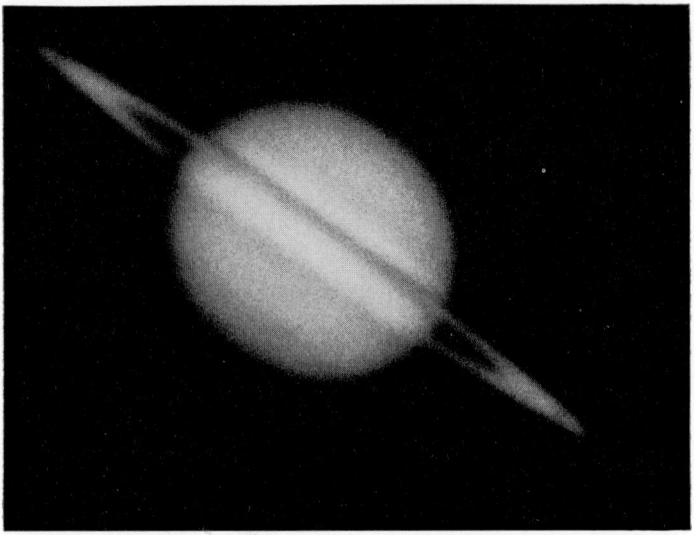

PLATE IV. Giant planet Saturn, rotating quickly, of very light constitution, with flat meteoritic rings, within zone where singular satellites cannot exist. (*Reproduction permission Pic du Midi.*)

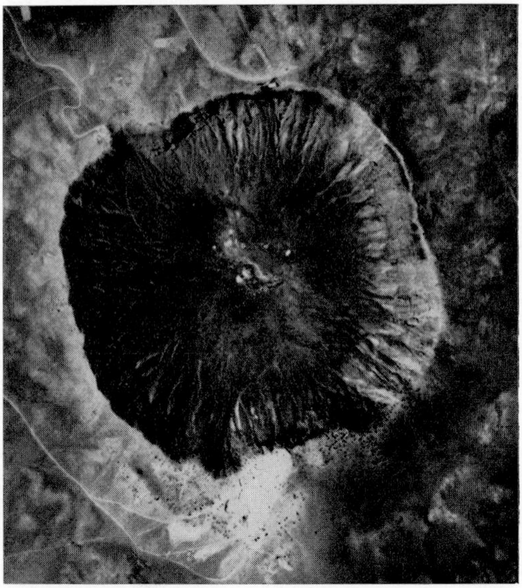

PLATE V. The Arizona impact crater, a rather recent relic, equivalent to many lunar craters, one of the rare survivors in a dry climate of terrestrial strong erosion.

required than is needed to precipitate a plane water layer. In the first case "super saturation" or "super cooling" is required. Moreover, nuclei of condensation facilitate the formation of small water drops in the air.

The same is true for the formation of small ice crystals, for instance those constituting cirrus clouds. In surroundings below freezing point, water vapour may condense directly into snow instead of into rain. However, this occurs also only at temperatures rather far below 0°C.

In the primeval nebula, apparently, the transformation of gases into liquids is very rare. The transformation of gases directly into solids, "sublimation", at sufficiently low temperatures is the only phenomenon that counts. Ter Haar, after a careful study of temperatures and densities in the primeval nebula, and the "sublimation heats" of different substances, could point out the almost certain existence of many kinds of small crystals in the solar nebula. But those in the region of the terrestrial planets consisted of metals and different types of inorganic compounds only; those in the region of the big planets consisted of combinations, such as cyanic acid, water, and ammonia.

38. Meteorites

IN CONSIDERING this subject we are reminded of the appearances of meteorites, a regular precipitation of cosmic grit and dust on the Earth. Most of these meteorites are so small that, when invading our atmosphere with velocities of 10, 20, 30 km/sec, they evaporate in the highest air layers.

Among meteorites there are, however, massive ones which actually drop down on to the Earth's surface. Many thousands of them have been found and chemically analysed.

A remarkable fact is the existence of two specific types of meteorites. We meet small grains up to large lumps, consisting mainly of iron and nickel, and those made of stony substances. One wonders whether this could be a freak of nature or could be related to the internal structure of the Earth, consisting as it does of an iron–nickel core and a stony mantle.

These two different classes of meteorites remain unintelligible unless we dare to assume with Urey and others that they have formed a part of larger bodies within which they were sorted out and not assembled. Such "parent bodies" would not be bigger than about the one-thousandth part of the Earth. The asteroids are examples of such bodies and collisions between asteroids, as was shown by Hirayama and D. Brouwer, must have happened in the recent past.

39. Comets

COMETS are swarms of meteorites, consisting of solid "ices", stone, and iron grains. These ices, besides water–ice, are carbonic acid–ice, cyanic–ice, methane–ice, and ammonia–ice. All these materials in the nuclei of comets, as long as these comets are moving far away in space, are frozen together, resulting in a composition reminding us strongly of the composition of the big planets, but without their hydrogen and helium.

When comets approach the Sun they are heated up, and vapours and dust are liberated from the meteorites. These substances constitute the tails of the comets. They are mostly absent from those meteorites that hit the Earth. The only substance these meteorites might perhaps bring down in measurable quantity is water.

Meteorites in empty space are lumps of ice with some iron and stony grit. But if it is true that lumps of ice and dust are formed spontaneously in empty space, are not they the proper building materials of the planets? Are planets, indeed, as propounded by Chamberlin and Moulton, collections of "planetesimals"? Almost certainly it is not without significance that planetesimals still continue to land on Earth and make it grow.

40. Saturn's Rings

THE second reason why we are asking the question of how the planets and satellites acquired their building materials with so much insistence, is that Saturn's ring consists of planetesimals. These small grains were identified by Kuiper as "hail stones". Is not this ring (Fig. 18) a satellite *in statu nascendi*, a prominent example, pointing out the course of development of satellites and therewith also the course of development of planets?

Now, at this point, we should be careful not to walk into a well-known trap, the mixing up of cause and effect. In any case there is positive ground for the existence of a ring around Saturn, even of rings, in the place of satellites. We have touched on this already when we indicated how the tidal force of a large body may threaten the existence of a small body in its near neighbourhood. Roche showed within what distance from the planet a satellite is in danger. If the mean density of a satellite is equal to the mean density of the planet, it circulates safely only at distances from the centre greater than 2·44 planet radii. When circulating within this range it is torn into pieces. The rings of Saturn, an inner light veil ring and an outer ring, which in fact consists of two bright rings separated by Cassini's dark division, are circulating between 1·15 and 2·26 times Saturn's radius. In spite of the minor uncertainties inherent in problems of this kind, we may say that in the region of the rings no satellite of larger dimension can ever have developed. In fact we do not find any there, whereas Janus circulates at a distance of 2·65 times the planet's radius, but if the satellites of Saturn, for instance, had experienced resistance in this planet's initial

60 *The Origin of the Solar System*

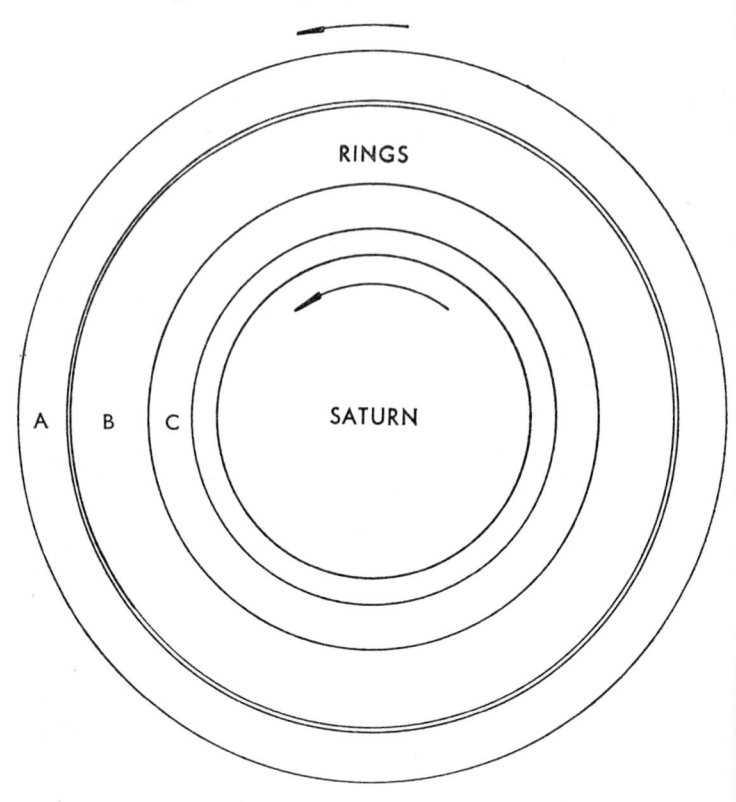

FIG. 18. Saturn's system of rings. Inwards: ring *A*, Cassini's division, ring *B*, and veil ring *C*. The radii are given in the right proportion.

hydrogen and helium envelope, and had been obliged to spiral inward, the inner satellites might have been destroyed when crossing the critical Roche's limit.

Now let us return to the possibilities and probabilities of condensation in the primeval nebula. In our terrestrial atmosphere we have the most obvious example of rain originating where water-vapour is subjected to supercooling. If water-vapour existed in the primeval nebula, and almost certainly it did in relatively large amounts, it must have existed beyond Mars in the form of small ice crystals. The material destined to form planets was present in the primeval nebula as gas or as snow.

However, the ice crystals probably did not grow so easily. They collided in the primeval nebula repeatedly, and because these collisions occurred between objects moving at high speeds, the crystals, as Hoyle was the first to point out, were subjected alternately to destruction and rebuilding. The primeval nebula will have consisted, on the one hand, of gases of which hydrogen, helium, and neon only were permanent throughout the solar system, and on the other of "smoke"—matter in the form of small solid particles of very different dimensions which may well be denoted as giant molecules. There is, however, an important contrast between the behaviour of dust and gas. Collisions between molecules are, except in limiting cases, elastic; collisions between dust particles are inelastic.

41. The Theoretical Structure of the Solar Nebula

WE ARE now in a position to consider what structure the primeval nebula will assume by its own forces.

Suppose, in the first instance, that the solar nebula is throughout gaseous. Let us further assume that the mean molecular weight of the prominent gases in a given region determines the constitution of a planet born in that region.

The Earth is built up for a large part out of substances such as iron and silicon-dioxide, whose molecular weights are 56 and 60, whereas Uranus and Neptune consist most probably of substances such as water, ammonia, and methane, whose molecular weights are 18, 17, and 16. A welcome circumstance, simplifying greatly our considerations, is that the local mean molecular weights and local gas temperatures are in such constant proportion that gas pressure p and gas density ρ are roughly in a constant proportion throughout the nebula.

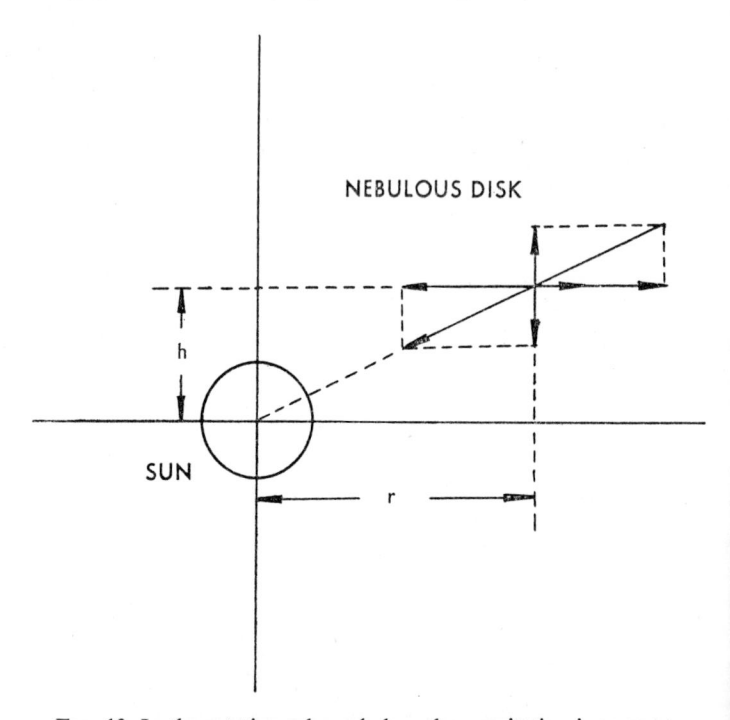

FIG. 19. In the rotating solar nebula, solar gravitation is compensated by pressure gradient and centrifugal force.

The balance of forces is shown by Fig. 19. In the spinning nebula, solar attraction is in equilibrium with the gradient of gas pressure and centrifugal force.

The simplicity of this equilibrium is due to the fact that the angular velocity ω of an element is independent of its height h above the equatorial plane. Thus the nebula rotates cylinderwise.

If ρ_e, the density of the gas in the equatorial plane at the distance r from the central axis, is constant,

$$\omega^2 r^3 = \text{constant}. \qquad (4)$$

This is Kepler's third law. Hence, in belts in which ρ_e increases with r, the angular velocity is higher than the velocity of a planet circulating at this distance from the centre, whereas in belts in which ρ_e decreases with r, the angular velocity is lower than the planet's velocity.

This is the time to deal with our assumption that internal friction has almost finished its work and has deformed the nebula to a semi-permanent flat structure, forced to move in nearly circular orbits about its central axis. If this had never been achieved, such a strictly ordered system of planets could never have been created.

If this is true, we may well try to answer the questions: Where does further natural transformation lead to? What is the structure of the primary nebula just before its last change of shape, its agglomeration into a family of planets? Viscosity, as we know, leads to conditions characterized by minimum loss of energy.

When this rule is applied, a meridional section through the nebula can be drawn. It is shown in the right half of Fig. 20.

The primeval disk did *not* show the lenticular shape one might have had in mind. The lines of equal density in the axial section represented here, show that the primeval disk was of a torus-like structure. An envelope marked 10^{-24} shows where the disk is merged into the interstellar medium. Within our region of the galaxy the interstellar material density amounts to a value of this order. The section through the envelope marked 10^{-22}, however, is also dotted, because it can hardly be counted as the actual envelope of the nebula. The surface 10^{-20} is the more reasonable envelope. A density of 10^{-18} g/cm^3 is reached

64 The Origin of the Solar System

in the terrestrial atmosphere at an altitude of 300 km, where modern missiles circulate safely, but where the air is dense enough to cause polar lights. Not before having experienced a density of the air of 10^{-16} g/cm³ meteorites flash up as "shooting stars". The surface 10^{-18} envelops Pluto's orbit, and arguments

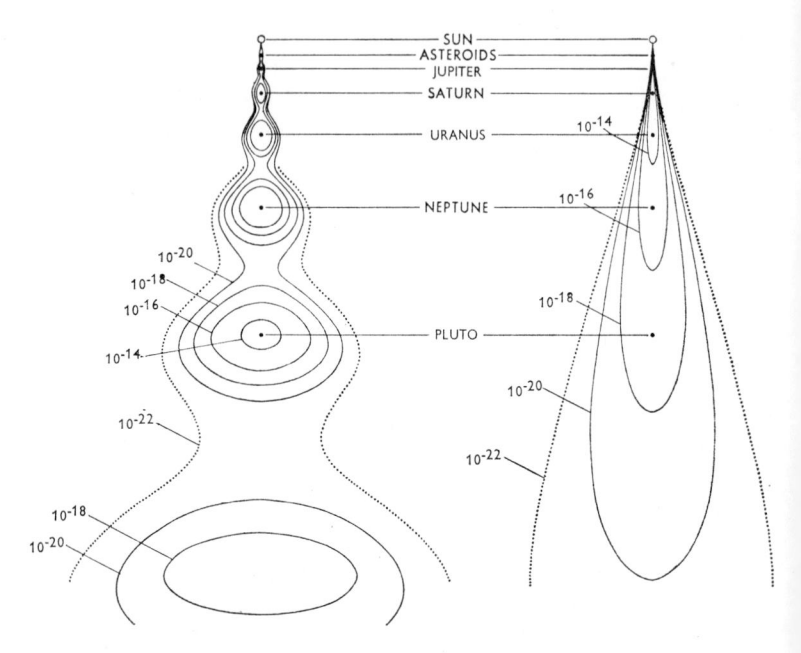

Fig. 20. One half of section through the solar nebula: (right) in quasi-steady rotation, and (left) at the start of the evolution of a set of rings leading to final condensation.

will be given for the thesis that the matter present between the surfaces 10^{-18} and 10^{-20} has served as the storehouse of comets. Within the surface 10^{-16} the regular planetary system originated, and the flatness of the primeval nebula, even up to this distance from the centre, is quite impressive.

As a matter of fact, Fig. 20 gives strong support to the hypothesis that the planetary system developed from a gas disk in quasi-steady motion.

42. The Solar Nebula a Cartesian Vortex as well as a Kantian Disk

IT IS fascinating to observe how rightly the solar nebula not only *may* be typified as a whirl in the interstellar medium, but also *must* be typified as such. Depending on the manner in which we view it, the solar nebula appears as a Cartesian vortex or as a Kantian disk.

Now the structure of the solar nebula has been so thoroughly discussed because almost all modern hypotheses on the origin of the planets start from the concept of this nebula and it is a good thing to have a basis which is no longer denied by anyone. However, as was mentioned earlier, with these considerations we have not yet advanced far. From this point on, different investigators have followed widely diverging paths.

How is this possible? If the nebula in its quasi-steady state is subjected to mathematical analysis, it should be possible to indicate the kind of further deformation the disk is likely to suffer.

43. From a Kantian Disk to Laplacean Rings

THE solar nebula was almost certainly destined to change shape from a disk to a series of concentric rings. Wishing to prove this, we should keep in mind the following basic theorem. When a mechanical equilibrium is disturbed, as is the case with a falling body, the tendency is towards a reduction in potential energy and an increase in kinetic energy. As will be mentioned later, Poincaré made use of this theorem in order to prove that the triaxial ellipsoid, which according to Jacobi is the equilibrium figure of a quickly rotating fluid mass, assumes the form of a pear when a given threshold value of the ratio of angular velocity to the density of the body is surpassed (see section 65).

Now it can be shown that when specific density waves (Fig. 21) are superimposed on the previous continuous decrease

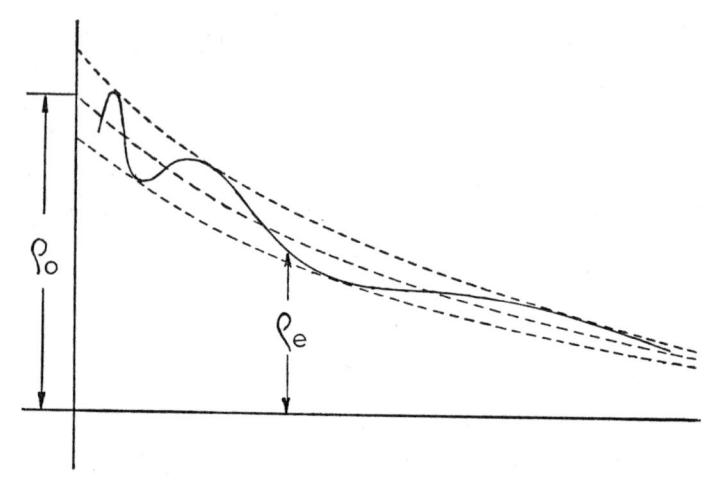

FIG. 21. The undulation on the radial decrease of the density in the equatorial plane where the disk strives after.

of the density in the equatorial plane ρ_e from the centre to the periphery of the disk, kinetic energy increases at the cost of potential energy. The disk assumes naturally sequences of circular ripples of this particular kind.

Whether or not a certain amount of the disk's kinetic energy is meanwhile transformed by internal friction into heat is of minor importance. The falling body just considered may reach the bottom and come to rest, heating the point of impact and growing hot itself. Here, however, lies the link between the theorem just cited and the theorem of minimum energy dissipation.

Suppose, for instance, the gas disk changes into a set of concentric rings; then the internal friction in the gas mass must have decreased because the rings are no longer rubbing the one against the other. The absolute minimum, zero energy dissipation, is finally reached when the rings are transformed into planets.

44. Strong Arguments for the Ring Phase

THE Russian astronomer O. J. Schmidt and the author, having reached the same conclusion along different paths, both gave strong support to a transformation of the disk, when gaseous, into a set of concentric rings following the rule

$$r_{n+1}^{\frac{1}{2}} - r_n^{\frac{1}{2}} = \text{constant.} \tag{5}$$

The variables r_{n+1} and r_n denote two successive ring radii. Consequently, the radii of the orbits of the planets, if they are condensation products of these rings, should follow the same rule.

Now the quite surprising fact is that the radii of the planetary orbits appear to do so, provided we restrict ourselves to the big planets and Pluto (Table 10). In this case there is no escape from

TABLE 10. SEQUENCE OF DISTANCES OF THE PLANETS FROM THE SUN

Distance (a.u.)	Pluto	Neptune	Uranus	Saturn	Jupiter	II	I
r	39·5	30·1	19·2	9·54	5·20		
Vr observed	6·29	5·48	4·38	3·09	2·28		
Vr assumed	6·28	5·28	4·28	3·28	2·28	1·28	0·28

the conclusion that the planetary system was created in two phases. In the first phase the four big planets and Pluto were assembled, a fifth big planet (II) at a distance of $1 \cdot 28^2$ or $1 \cdot 64$ a.u., and possibly a small planet (I) very close to the Sun. The big planet II was evidently never completed. The set of terrestrial planets came in its place.

TABLE 11. PLANETARY MASSES, THEORETICAL AND OBSERVED, IN EARTH MASSES

Pluto	Neptune	Uranus	Saturn	Jupiter	II	I
0·8	5·9	35·4	133	271	122	1·5
0·05	17·6	14·5	95	317		

Following these indications the masses of the planets should have attained the values shown in Table 11. The general distribution of the masses of the planets appears naturally, from the centre towards the periphery, first as an increase, then a decrease in the masses of the planets. This variation is produced because the matter available to form a planet is gathered from a belt whose dimension is outwardly increasing, whereas the density of the matter within each belt is outwardly decreasing. This principle will not disappoint us once we have accepted the theory of the disk.

Planet I would have originated very near the Sun. It remained, if conceived at all, probably in the ring phase and was finally united with the Sun. Planet II would have obtained a mass of 122 earth masses. Hence the total mass of materials available to this planet would have exceeded the mass of all terrestrial planets together by about 50 times. These proportions are not surprising. The hydrogen and the helium might have moved from the centre to the periphery of the solar nebula before the other heavier substances were able to assemble and give birth to the terrestrial planets. This phase of development may, therefore, be considered separately. Moreover, we notice that the terrestrial planets themselves follow the same distance rule remarkably well (Table 12). Even the distribution of the masses is similar. From the centre towards the periphery they at first increase and then decrease.

TABLE 12. SEQUENCE OF DISTANCES OF THE PLANETS FROM THE SUN

Distance (a.u)	Asteroids	Mars	Earth	Venus	Mercury
r		1·52	1·00	0·72	0·29
Vr observed		1·23	1·00	0·85	0·62
Vr assumed	1·42	1·22	1·02	0·82	0·62

Finally, we can hardly escape the conclusion that the asteroids belong to the group of terrestrial planets and play in this group the part of the little and irregular Pluto in the main group.

45. Can we Explain the Rule of Titius and Bode?

THE hypothesis sketched above makes a promising impression, and there is no objection against following the view of a creation of the planetary system in two phases. When the author nevertheless became the supporter of a minimum number of hypotheses *ad hoc* and of a creation of the planetary system in one continuous act, it was because the accumulation of molecular matter to meteoritic particles and the inelastic collisions between these particles were not only essential, but also provided sufficient conditions for the evolution of the planetary system from the solar nebula. It is necessary not only that sufficient internal energy is stored up in a given ring, but also that this internal energy becomes available in the course of the ring's development. To achieve this the particles of the ring have to collide and group together. Consequently, kinetic energy is lost and potential energy released by a certain approach of the ring's mass towards the centre of the system.

Let us add that the rings are not formed synchronously, but in succession, their formation being started by the first one that is going to condense and generate a planet. We shall later see who that first-born probably was.

As regards temperature, it is sufficient to distinguish the following three cases:

(a) uniform temperature;
(b) solar nebula in radiative equilibrium with the Sun;
(c) solar nebula in conditions of maximum stability.

In these three cases the following particular rules of planetary distances from the Sun apply:

$$r_{n+1} - r_n = \text{constant}, \qquad (6)$$

$$r_{n+1}^{\frac{1}{2}} - r_n^{\frac{1}{2}} = \text{constant}, \qquad (7)$$

$$r_{n+1} : r_n = \text{constant}. \qquad (8)$$

These variations on the classical theme of "the harmony of the spheres" are illustrative. Provided the solar nebula starts from conditions of maximum stability, the radii of the orbits of the planets will follow a geometric series. Provided the solar nebula was in radiative equilibrium with the Sun, we meet the relation derived earlier. It applies to the four terrestrial planets and the asteroids, and to the four major planets and Pluto separately, with outstanding precision.

Now, only relation (8) can be approximately valid throughout one system from its centre to its periphery. It is therefore illuminating to observe how the planetary system, by its partition into two groups, not only supports this argument, but also supports the hypothesis that the solar nebula was dominantly gaseous and in radiative equilibrium with the Sun.

The case $n = 0$, implying uniform temperature throughout the solar nebula, is obviously irrelevant.

The fact that Ter Haar and others could so well explain the different constitutions of the terrestrial and the major planets as being due to the different ways of condensation of their basic solid particles in regions of different temperature, does not contradict in any way our present conclusion. In the solar nebula "sedimentation" of particulate matter towards the equatorial plane must have occurred. Each planet passed through a stage, which was rightly distinguished by Kuiper as a "sediment ring".

46. The Masses of the Planets to a First Approximation

IF MATERIAL equal to the total mass of the planets is supposed to have been available in the solar nebula, and if the geometric series for the radii of the planetary orbits is accepted, transformation of the solar nebula would lead to masses of the planets, as presented in Table 13.

TABLE 13. THE MASSES OF THE PLANETS IN EARTH MASSES

	Theoretical	Observed
Mercury	0·71	0·05
Venus	3·24	0·81
Earth	12·7	1
Mars	30·5	0·11
Asteroids	87·2	—
Jupiter	133	317
Saturn	118	95
Uranus	51·4	14·5
Neptune	8·6	17·6
Pluto	0·4	0·05?

It is interesting to see how far the present theory of the creation of our planetary system extends, even without the application of the slight corrections which are probably required.

In the first place the variation with distance from the Sun of the masses of the planets is interpreted correctly. Jupiter is, both in fact and theory, the heaviest planet. Moreover, it is interesting to note that we can hardly expect one more planet beyond Pluto. Such a planet, if it ever originated, would have been so small as to remain invisible. However, whether Pluto is single or perhaps the biggest member of an outer swarm of "planetoids" is open for discussion. Are we going to distinguish in future the "plutoids", playing beyond the big planets the part that the "planetoids" play beyond the terrestrial planets?

47. The Outer Limit of the Solar System

WE SHOULD, however, consider the evolution of Pluto from another point of view. The extremely low density of the gas or the dust in the solar nebula where Pluto moves and the immense volume of the ring, supposed to be concentrated into this planet, suggest that the agglomeration of matter might perhaps have permitted the formation of a swarm of meteorites and comets. But the creation of Pluto, a planet as big as Mercury, must have been extremely improbable. We shall have to come back to Pluto—one of the celestial bodies, about which mystery still hangs (see section 71).

Returning to Table 13 we notice that the terrestrial planets probably got hold of much less matter than was theoretically in store for them. About 90 per cent of the lighter substances were lost by these planets, while Mars must have lost by far the greater part and the asteroids, almost the total amount of matter concentrated in their rings.

Further Adjustment of the Theory and what Results from this 73

Was this surplus matter lost to the greedy Jupiter, already the biggest mass? Jupiter must certainly have become the most important disturber of the "nest of ants", the belt of innumerable asteroids. Did no more than a handful of marbles remain from the previous multitude of grains?

48. Further Adjustment of the Theory and what Results from this

IT IS possible to fit these arguments more carefully in our picture. The whole picture is perhaps the composition of a number of primitive pictures. The evolution from disk to rings may well have started with the appearance of more than one set of ripples, just like the different kinds we can find moving along a disturbed water surface at one time. If the approximation is made in the best possible way, Table 14 results.

TABLE 14.

| | Log_{10} distance (Earth = 1) || Mass ||
	Assumed	Observed	Calculated	Observed
Within	−1·255		0·0002	
orbit of	−1·004		0·07	
Mercury	−0·753		0·07	
Mercury	−0·502	−0·412	0·04	0·05
Venus	−0·251	−0·144	0·83	0·81
Earth	0	0	1	1
Mars	0·251	0·183	0·11	0·11
Asteroids	0·502	—	2·57	Very small
Jupiter	0·753	0·716	309	317
Saturn	1·004	0·980	98	95
Uranus	1·255	1·283	13·5	14·5
Neptune	1·506	1·478	18·6	17·6
Pluto	1·757	1·596	0·2	0·05 ?
Beyond Pluto	2·008		0·00003	

Now it would be unfair to point out the remarkable success exhibited in the excellent agreement between the observed and calculated masses of the planets. What we did was to approximate as closely as possible the actual variation of the masses of the planets from the centre to the periphery of the system with the aid of two radial density waves, which both may have transformed the primeval disk, and to reconstruct the original variation by applying the amplitudes and lengths of the waves derived. Nevertheless, more was gained by this operation than superficially appears. We can prove that the radial density waves, superimposed on the fundamental radial density wave leading to separate planets, show amplitudes of a smaller order of magnitude than the primary one. Consequently, the masses of the planets may show rather large deviations from their "normal" values, such as are revealed by the contrast of Jupiter to Mars, although the planets remain bound to follow closely the fundamental rule of distances, viz. the geometric series.

We may draw another conclusion from Table 14. Two planets within the orbit of Mercury and acquiring masses exceeding the mass of Mercury, might have come into existence. It is obvious, however, that solar tidal forces and the very high temperature of the gas in the near neighbourhood of the Sun may have prevented their formation. Mercury, by its unusually large eccentricity and orbital inclination, indicates that the outstanding regularity in the planetary system was due to fail at shorter distances from the Sun.

On the other hand, nobody should cherish illusions about the discovery of a transplutonian planet. For the creation of a single planet of any importance beyond Pluto no adequate quantity of matter has ever been available.

A third remarkable point is that theory supplies a value for the mass of a planet between Mars and Jupiter, assuming that no disturbances prevented its agglomeration. The mass of this "virtual" planet amounts to $2 \cdot 57$ earth masses, viz. a mass between those of the Earth and Uranus. This planet and its disappearance provide enough material for a "detective story".

49. The Mean Densities of Planets and Satellites

BEFORE entering upon the question of the origin of the asteroids, let us review the mean densities of the bodies of the solar system. What has become known today is contained in one graph, Fig. 22. It gives the mean density in g/cm³ of the members of the solar family as a function of the logarithm of their masses, the mass of the Earth having been taken as unit.

The dots have been assembled in strips. Uncertain dots are question marked. It should be remembered in particular that Eros and Ceres are two asteroids whose masses and diameters have been estimated only.

The satellites of Jupiter, whose masses, diameters and mean densities are adequately known, are the four Galileians: Io, Europa, Ganymede, and Callisto. The detailed investigations of the mutual perturbations between the satellites of Saturn made by W. de Sitter and G. Struve, permitted a reliable determination of the masses and densities of most of them. We meet in sequence, from the centre to the periphery of their system, Mimas, Enceladus, Thetys, Dione, Rhea, Titan, Hyperion, and Japetus. We have to know more about Janus before entering it in the present scheme. Triton is a remarkably large satellite of Neptune.

When looking at the graph from left to right, that is from the smaller to the larger masses, we experience, so to speak, the accumulation of all these bodies out of planetesimals. Moreover, we have to take into account the compression that causes the density of the massive bodies to be greater than the density of their material under normal conditions. Increasing temperature will expand almost all matter, one of the noteworthy exceptions being water–ice, and eventually change it from the solid state to the liquid state and then to the gaseous state, or directly from the solid state to the gaseous state. This latter transition and its reverse is called "sublimation", and it is the only process that counts in the interplanetary rarified medium.

50. The Chemical Composition of Planets and Satellites

THE graph presented in Fig. 22 starts from the left with bodies divided in two clearly separated density classes. The lowest path leads along the exceptionally light satellites of Saturn, which evidently get denser by compression with the growth of their masses, viz. Mimas, Enceladus, Thetys, Japetus, and Rhea. We are inclined to doubt the reliability of the density of Dione, as it should be closer to $1 \cdot 8$ than to $2 \cdot 8$.

The middle path leads along densities which are typical for "stony meteorites" and the Moon. The Moon's density is $3 \cdot 3$. Although the density values of Eros, Hyperion, and Ceres are doubtful, this line rises regularly with the compression for the greater masses. The group Europa, Io, Moon, opens, in a sense, the route of the planets. It rises further along Mars and Mercury towards Venus and the Earth. The latter three planets reach the highest mean density. The position of little Mercury leads to the interesting conclusion that iron and nickel must have been concentrated towards the Sun before the solar nebula condensed into planets.

The Chemical Composition of Planets and Satellites

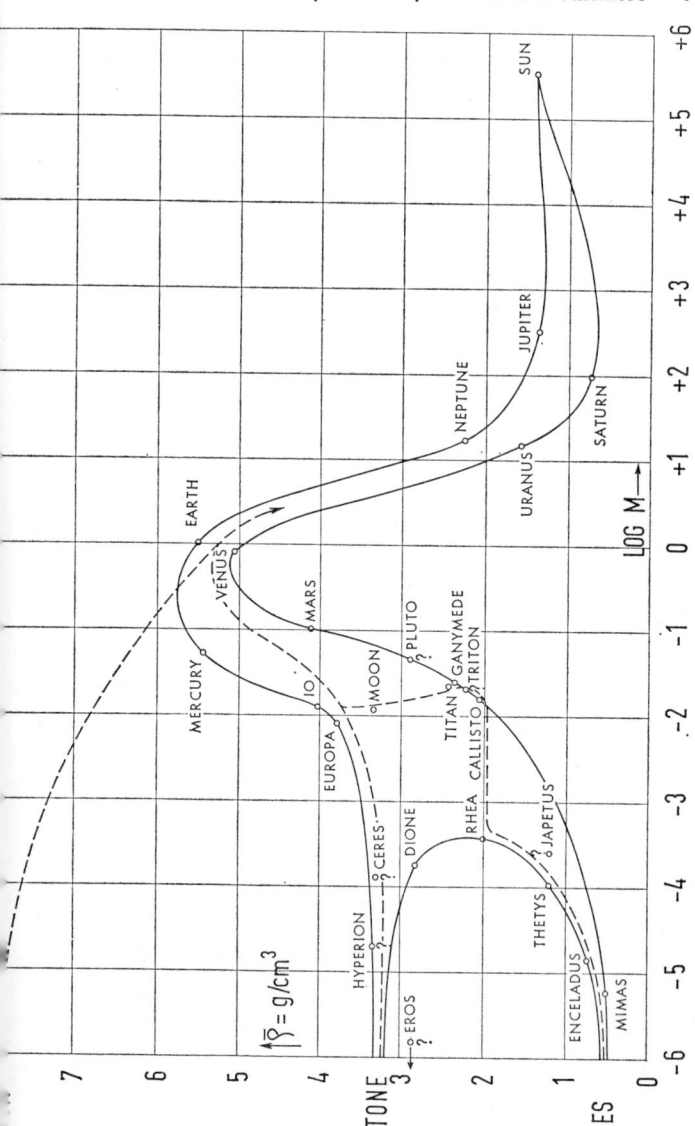

FIG. 22. The characteristic dependence of the mean density of the bodies of the solar system on their masses. The masses are given in logarithmic measure, the mass of the Earth being taken as unit.

78   The Origin of the Solar System

This progression of densities suggests strongly that the three characteristic groups of substances enumerated in Table 15 all take part in the structure of the planets and their satellites. The substances of the upper group, all liquid or solid at the

TABLE 15. DENSITIES OF SOME FLUID AND SOLID SUBSTANCES OF IMPORTANCE IN COSMOGONY

	Molecular weight	Density in (g/cm^3)	
		Fluid	Solid
Methane	16	0·42	
Ammonia	17	0·60	0·82
Water	18	1·00	0·92
Silicon-dioxide	60		2·65
Magnesium-oxide	40		3·22
Ferrous-sulphite	88		4·84
Iron	56	7·23	7·86
Nickel	58	8·79	8·90

distance from the Sun where Saturn circulates, have evidently contributed to the formation of the minor satellites of Saturn. These substances are the diverse "ices" mentioned earlier (see section 39).

Water–ice as one of the main constituents of these satellites is not excluded. The grains in the rings of Saturn are probably "hail stones". The "ices" under high compression reach perhaps densities of about 2, a value approached frequently. Yet it is possible and even probable that in all bodies whose density is about 2 a small percentage of substances with densities of about 3, 4, and 5 under normal conditions, are also present.

Titan, Ganymede, Callisto, and Triton are grouped so tightly together that they evidently mark a typical phase in the agglomeration of members of the solar system. Have these members perhaps grown so far that water has started to evaporate and leave the body? Does the pock-marked face of our Moon express, perhaps, besides bombardments, an intense activity of "fumaroles"? In any case the Moon is on the evolutionary route from Titan and Ganymede towards Europa and Io. If this is true, the water should have left the latter two satellites. The Moon still possesses perhaps a significant quantity of water in its interior, whereas Europa and Io consist almost exclusively of the substances of the middle group. We meet these satellites on the "assembly line" from the smaller bodies with a density of over 3 to the terrestrial planets with higher densities.

Evidently the "iron meteorites" enter the scheme along the third route with densities 7 to 8. They represent very probably the building materials of the cores of the terrestrial planets, those of Mercury, Venus, and the Earth, and possibly also, to a lesser degree, the core of Mars.

Continuing our way along Venus and the Earth the density curve dives down straight to Neptune and Uranus. Jupiter and Saturn with greater mass and still lower density come next. Finally, the average density curve ascends again slightly and terminates in the Sun at the 1·4 level.

It is clear that in the "cascade" the lighter substances out of the three characteristic groups are going to preponderate, while finally the upperhand is gained by those substances which were not distinguished here, hydrogen and helium. When all this is considered, the graph is a revelation.

Pluto cannot contain hydrogen and helium in important quantity. Consequently it is probably a rather small planet whose density is at most 3 — a density which may be designated as the standard density of those celestial bodies consisting mainly of substance of the middle group.

51. Is there an Unfinished or Exploded Planet between Mars and Jupiter?

WHAT should be thought of the curious fate of the planet with a mass of 2 to 3 earth masses, which should have taken the place of the asteroids?

Figure 22 shows us that the position of this planet in the heart of the "cascade" must have been dangerous. During its condensation the temperature of the relatively small planet increased probably so much that it was not able to retain its evaporating constituents. It is still far from clear what exactly happened. Did the planet explode, a possibility suggested by Ramsey and Lighthill, or was it broken up while contracting? The most plausible view is that the planet's assemblage was never completed. In any case Urey and other investigators assure us that meteorites cannot have been built up in strong gravitational fields. On the other hand, meteorites are not likely to be free agglomerations either, and for their formation require "parent bodies" of asteroid size.

Now, as we know, relatively heavy asteroids have been split up into swarms of lighter asteroids. Their common source is still traceable. Consequently, collisions between asteroids must have occurred at rather recent dates.

What has actually been the fate of all this grit and dust? The total mass of the present asteroids is so small that almost all these bodies must have been dispersed. How and whither?

52. The Coming and Going of Comets

EVER since the discovery of the asteroids the problem of their dispersal has been studied, and the great disturber of the "nest of ants" proved to be Jupiter.

The well-known Jovian family of comets also indicated connections of this kind. There have never been reasons to attribute to any meteorite the velocity which would be reached by starting far out in space with a finite velocity in the direction of the Sun.

Strömgren pointed out that the comets, which are the suppliers of our swarms of meteorites, are practically all members of the solar system. They are moving in highly eccentric but elliptic orbits. In those few cases of apparent disagreement, one of the big planets, in particular the giant Jupiter, could be shown to have thrown the comet from an elliptic into a hyperbolic orbit—one of no return.

But how is it possible that a comet approaching the Sun again and again loses some matter by evaporation of its lighter substances, which, as Whipple plausibly indicated, were previously bound together with dust, grit, and stones? A comet never returns to its region of origin in the same condition as it was during its appearance near the Sun. Comets are slowly degenerating. Even a specimen like Halley's, which returns only once in every 76 years, has evidently lost part of the brightness it had at its earliest appearance, recorded by the Chinese in 240 B.C. Where is this distant store of comets located?

Oort gave a striking answer to this question. A store of comets exists in the form of a cloud, some ten thousands of astronomical units in size, enveloping the solar system. Foreign stars, when moving through the cloud, perturb the comets and direct them into new orbits. Some of them by chance pass near the Sun and are then stored away again, with the exception of those few comets which, under the influence of planetary perturbations, become periodic.

Now this immense cloud of comets poses the fascinating question: How did it originate? Large numbers of comets, or else, swarms of meteorites were apparently collected along the periphery of the solar nebula, whereas its central portion condensed into planets. There are, however, serious objections against the thesis that all meteorites originated in that extremely rarified outer portion of the nebula. Where would they have obtained their iron from? The outer portion of the nebula must have consisted almost exclusively of the lighter substances and hydrogen and helium, supplying materials for the big planets. Even when looking from the periphery to the centre of the solar system we can hardly expect before Saturn a large core of terrestrial rocks, and hardly before Jupiter a small core of iron.

53. Is the Ring of Asteroids Dispersed?

THUS attention is drawn to the ring of asteroids as the source of comets. It would have been Jupiter, the giant planet, who rampaged most strongly among the asteroids. This planet's disturbing forces have often been given as the reason for the next "planetary ring" within Jupiter's orbit never having condensed into one planet. Most probably the present swarm of asteroids is only an extremely small remnant of the total mass of the materials assembled in the ring of the asteroids in its earliest state.

Oort estimates that Jupiter's perturbations transferred one-thirtieth of this mass into the cloud of comets, whereas the rest of this mass escaped completely or dropped into the Sun. If the author's estimate of the original total mass of the asteroids is right, about eight-hundredths of the Earth's mass should have been available to form the cloud of comets. Oort estimates the total mass of all comets in the cloud to be three-hundredths of the Earth's mass. These two amounts are so similar that every experienced investigator in the present field will inquire where a mistake was made, since he is not used to finding hypotheses so well verified quantitatively.

54. Radiation Pressure, Poynting–Robertson Effect, and Zodiacal Light

WE HAVE to indicate, finally, another dispersing force experienced by small dust particles circulating round the Sun. The ring of asteroids, especially in its most refined condition, must have been largely influenced by this force.

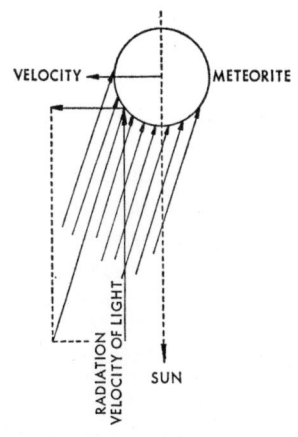

FIG. 23. The Poynting–Robertson effect of solar radiation pressure on the motion of a meteorite.

Robertson was the first to point out this effect. It was derived from Poynting's study of the electromagnetic theory of light and can be described as follows (Fig. 23): just as a walker in the rain gets more wet on his front than on his back, each small globe circulating round the sun receives more solar radiation on the hemisphere directed forward than on the hemisphere directed backward. A quantity of radiation represents a certain amount of energy and a certain amount of energy represents, according to general relativity, a certain amount of mass. Consequently, radiation possesses momentum and exercises pressure on a body receiving it. This pressure is known as "radiation pressure".

Now when radiation hits a meteorite a little more strongly on its front than on its back, that is more strongly in a direction opposite to the direction of motion of the meteorite, it is continuously slowed down. It will spiral in towards the Sun and finally fall into it.

The smaller the meteorite, the quicker its fall towards the Sun. The Poynting–Robertson effect on planets of normal size is negligibly small. However, Whipple could prove that all grains smaller than 1 mm travel down to the Sun from a distance of 5 a.u. in a time shorter than 1000 million years. The mass of dust falling down on Earth as cosmic dust is estimated to be a thousand times larger than the mass falling down as meteorites. However, it has become almost equally certain that the glimmer known as zodiacal light is due to a dust disk that is slowly shrinking and uniting with the Sun. Moreover, if embryos of planets once existed inside Mercury's orbit, these apparently united with the Sun in their dust-ring state. Hence, in order to explain the permanency of the zodiacal light, it must be assumed that there is a regular supply of materials to the solar nebula from outside. We can also see in the present disk the faint remains of the primeval disk bearing the planetary system. It is extremely instructive how so many seemingly unrelated phenomena fuse together into one homogeneous picture.

There are, however, two facets of this problem which oblige us to treat it with great care. Dust particles, of dimensions differing only slightly from sunlight wavelengths, are blown away from the Sun by "radiation pressure". For particles of molecular dimensions this radiation pressure has only slight significance. The reason is that an atom absorbs from solar radiation only the small part indicated by the Fraunhofer spectral lines connected with this particular atom. For the same reason the Poynting–Robertson effect on gas molecules is negligibly small.

Now, we should recognize the difficulty that both radiation pressure and the Poynting–Robertson effect may have intervened at some stage of the transformation of the solar dust disk into the set of concentric dust rings. However, the accretion of dust particles into grains and larger meteorites is probably achieved rather quickly, and hence the shortness of the critical interval may well have reduced the harm done by the two effects in the regular evolution of the planetary system. Moreover, the existence of satellite systems justifies our theory, since in their evolution the two effects can never have played any serious part.

55. Large-scale Turbulence Again

THE author has not concealed his distrust of the idea that any essential contribution was made by large-scale turbulence to the formation of the planetary system. However, he wishes to raise here some new objections against the hypothesis that turbulence played a major part.

In the first place it has been popular to consider the eddies as the units destined to be concentrated. In the primeval nebula, as in every liquid, eddies are in fact remarkably persistent units, but centrifugal force will reduce rather than increase the tendency for them to be concentrated by internal attraction. Moreover, how puzzling is the order in the planetary distances from the Sun, when contrasted with the disorder turbulence creates, when it does *not* lead to large cellular eddies as suggested by von Weizsäcker. Too often this order has been obscured.

An intricate aspect is the following. As the angular velocity in the nebula decreases from the centre to the periphery, each eddy shows a sense of rotation contrary to its sense of revolution round the Sun. The initial rotation of each "protoplanet" that is a direct condensation product of an eddy, would be in the wrong direction.

Only one answer has been given to the question of how protoplanets could have reversed their axial rotation, and this again leads us back to tidal forces.

56. Is the "Inversion" of the Axial Rotation of the Protoplanets an Effect of Solar Tidal Forces?

CONSIDER again a pair of celestial bodies of different class, a star with one planet or a planet with one satellite, the two globes circulating round their common centre of gravity. Bulges develop at both ends of the diameter of the secondary body directed towards the primary body. If the secondary body rotates around its axis, the tidal bulges are dragged around in the direction of rotation. As this drag can only be partly realized, the tidal bulges remain in a certain fixed position. The diameter connecting them makes a fixed angle with the diameter directed to the primary body. This angle plays an important role in the theory of tides. Experience, for instance, shows that the flood caused by the moontide occurs after the Moon has passed through the meridian at the place of observation, i.e. the two events are not synchronous.

During this process the tidal bulges stand still, whereas the globe on which they are raised rotates. This is never a strictly frictionless process. Consequently the tidal bulges act like brakes on the spinning globe. The process proceeds in a slightly different way on our Earth. In fact, flood-hills and ebb-valleys move around as surface waves over the oceans and the question arises as to what causes the braking influence of the tides. Now the movement of the tidal waves is at a forced speed. Moreover, tidal currents move twice a day in one direction and twice a day in the reverse direction through shallow seas and narrow straits. These currents in particular cause the tidal friction. It is not important to know how and where the tidal currents move. The braking action on the spinning Earth essentially amounts to a loss of energy. The lost energy is derived from the rotational energy of the Earth, and hence the rotation of the Earth is continuously slowed down.

A decrease in the speed of rotation is experienced by all celestial bodies subject to tidal forces. It depends wholly on the structure of the celestial body. The Earth is a solid body covered by oceans. In a completely solid body or in a completely liquid or gaseous body the internal friction due to the rhythmic deformation of the body has the same effect, although it is perhaps less efficient. The final result is that the satellite turns one and the same hemisphere towards its planet, or the planet one and the same hemisphere towards its parent star. Examples of such fixation are those of our Moon relative to the Earth and of Mercury and Venus relative to the Sun. Why the periods of rotation of Mercury and Venus show significant deviations from the strict rule, discovered recently—as was mentioned in section 2—is receiving great attention.

The tidal action between the two celestial bodies is reciprocal. However, the effect on the secondary body is stronger and quicker than the effect on the primary body. Hence a protoplanet experiences strong tidal actions from the Sun. Were perhaps all protoplanets obliged to present relatively quickly, one and the same hemisphere towards the Sun? What would this signify? The most important result is that the secondary body rotates in the same sense as it revolves round the primary body. The periods of axial rotation and of revolution are then equal.

Each contraction of a body accelerates its rotation. If protoplanets contracted, they would, as a matter of fact, start rotating in the same sense as their revolution round the Sun.

There are, however, serious objections against this simple

solution of a major problem. In the first place, why should the decelerating action of the tidal forces on a developing planet gain the upper hand over the accelerating action of the contraction? Moreover, the axes of most planets show the required tendency to a perpendicular position, but what shall we think of Uranus? It spoils the game. Uranus and its four big satellites are a prominent example of systematic structure. These four big satellites, Ariel, Umbriel, Titania, and Oberon, move in almost perfect circular orbits showing no measurable inclination relative to the planet's equator. Nevertheless, the inclination of the common axis of rotation relative to the ecliptic does not exceed 8°.

The hypothesis that proto-Uranus, by the braking action of tidal forces, reached a state of rest relative to the Sun and was accelerated thereafter fails completely. The author is convinced that the "tidal theory" of the axial rotation of the planets must be rejected. Hence, along this sidetrack we return to the theory of the concentric rings. Did we not prove that if the matter of one ring unites, the resulting body will rotate around an axis showing a strong tendency towards a perpendicular position in the orthodox sense?

How strictly are these tendencies realized? The inclinations of the equators of the planets to their orbital planes are as follows:

Mercury	—	Jupiter	$3 \cdot 1°$
Venus	—	Saturn	$26 \cdot 7°$
Earth	$23 \cdot 5°$	Uranus	$98 \cdot 0°$
Mars	$25 \cdot 2°$	Neptune	$29°$

The tendency of the axes of rotation towards a perpendicular position is only moderately strong, but beyond any doubt "statistically significant". Moreover why should we wonder about the rather large deviations of the axes of rotation from a perpendicular position? We considered only the "ideal" case, viz. that before their agglomeration the last and second last separate condensation products of an initial ring move in one and the same orbit. This, of course, can never have happened strictly. If the orbital planes of the final two coalescing parts of the ring did *not* exactly coincide, the conditions for a certain inclination of the equator of the resulting protoplanet to its orbital plane are satisfied. Even the position of Uranus and its satellite system is not surprising. Proto-Uranus may easily have ended in its remarkable position due to some random, unfavourable asymmetry.

We have now reached the point where we may repeat what we stated when reviewing the structure of the primeval solar nebula: the most puzzling problem arises not before, but after the formation of the embryo. The problem is this: How is a system of satellites to be created out of a disk in quasi-steady motion round a planet, this motion being in the same direction as the planet's rotation?

57. The Process of Condensation of Planetary Rings

OUR main example, the transformation of a nebular disk spinning round the Sun into a set of concentric planetary rings, can be studied in rather greater detail.

An arbitrary density wave, superimposed on the initial radial density distribution throughout the disk, will be intensified under specific conditions. The question is to what value must the amplitude of this density wave, say ϵ in a practical logarithmic measure, increase in order that a planetary ring will tend towards condensation. How large is the "critical" amplitude ϵ_c?

Roche's theory indicates the following values of ϵ_c, tabulated against r, the distance from the Sun.

90 The Origin of the Solar System

$r =$ cm	ϵ_c
10^{12}	14·9
10^{13}	7·3
10^{14}	7·2
10^{15}	15·0

ϵ_c shows a very flat minimum amounting to $7\cdot15$ at $r = 7\cdot74 \times 10^{13}$ cm. This distance is very near Jupiter's distance from the Sun. It thus becomes very probable that condensation started near Jupiter and proceeded from Jupiter towards Mercury on the one side, where $\epsilon_c = 10\cdot6$, and towards Neptune on the other side, where $\epsilon_c = 10\cdot3$. The critical density of the gas ρ_c which has to be exceeded in a "density ridge" if a planet is to condense there, is greatest near Mercury. The amount reached there is

$$\rho_c = 3\cdot50 \times 10^{-5} \text{ g/cm}^3.$$

To fix our ideas: this critical density of the gas is 40 times smaller than the density of our atmosphere near the Earth's surface.

In the adjacent "density troughs" the density then is of the order 10^{-14} g/cm^3. This shows us how far the development towards individual rings has proceeded before the critical phase starts. If the value $\epsilon_c = 8$ may be assumed to represent average conditions, then Fig. 20 (left part) shows us how a meridional section of the nebula looked in the beginning. Figure 24 represents a top view in rough outline.

An interesting point is relevant here. The "critical" amplitude of the density undulation reaches equal values near Mercury and Neptune. Hence, ϵ_c may perhaps have reached the value 11, but would not have exceeded it. For this reason no planets came into being inside Mercury or outside Neptune. The condensation reached in these parts of the disk did not allow further agglomeration. This would induce us to doubt the "genuineness" of Pluto as an independent planet.

What strikes us also is that the tendency towards condensation of the disk into planets was rather uniform, even between

The Process of Condensation of Planetary Rings 91

such extremes as Mercury and Neptune. This uniformity is evidently associated with the equilibrium conditions of the nebulous disk. The same consideration induced Kuiper to conclude that if the total mass of the nebula was sufficiently large, say, one-tenth of the solar mass, the density nearly everywhere would approach the critical limit of the density pointed out by Roche.

But it should be realized that we have avoided one major difficulty. It remains unproven that if agglomeration started

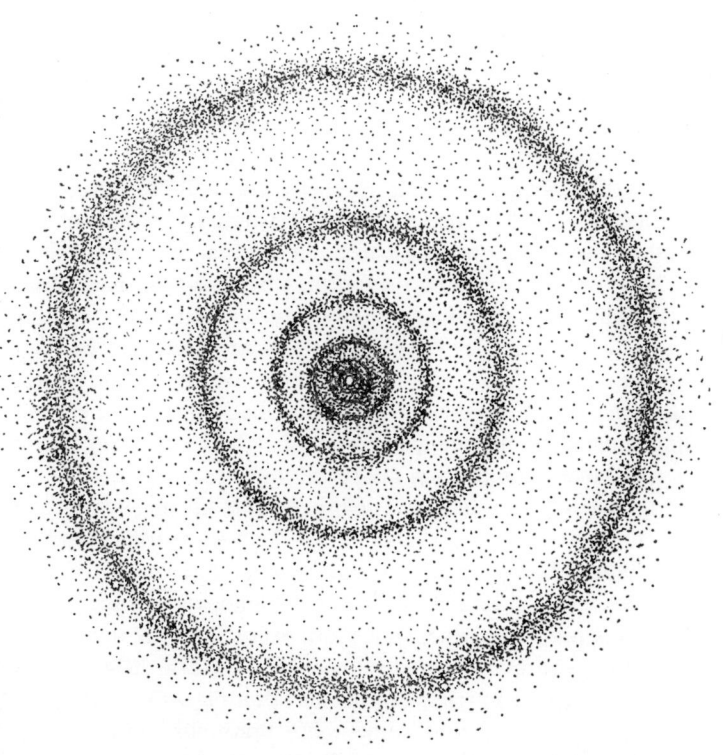

FIG. 24. Natural resolution of a nebulous disk into a set of concentric rings.

somewhere in the disk, for instance with Jupiter, the birth of other planets would not be prevented. Is it true that the disk, in consequence of the assemblage of materials into that first planet, was not deformed too much to allow similar agglomerations?

Let us try to answer this question after first having answered two other questions. The first of these questions is, whether in the critical stage described here the kinetic energy of the system could still grow at the cost of its potential energy. Now there is no serious reason for doubt because it can be shown that the final set of condensed globes possesses more kinetic energy than the primeval nebula. The next question is whether the motion of the gas or dust would perhaps become turbulent before the point of condensation is reached.

The radial variation of the angular velocity of the spinning disk—the quantity deciding whether there shall or shall not be turbulence—is itself dependent on the radial variation of the gas density. Consequently, a second critical amplitude ϵ_c exists.

Now we can draw two important conclusions. The initial disk would be and would remain in turbulent motion without showing any tendency towards condensation at distances from the Sun larger than $5 \cdot 31 \times 10^{15}$ cm, that is far beyond Pluto. However, when the disk is in transformation, the two critical limits just distinguished become equal at $3 \cdot 02 \times 10^{14}$ cm, that is at a distance from the Sun not far beyond Uranus. There, both limits reach the value $8 \cdot 9$. This proves that all rings may have remained stable with the exception of the rings bearing Neptune and Pluto. These rings reached the limit inducing turbulent motion before they reached the limit inducing condensation. Consequently, Neptune and Pluto were both in danger of remaining swarms of planetesimals. Neptune evidently escaped this danger, Pluto perhaps not. This latter planet's "eccentric" behaviour suggests that some more "plutoids" might exist. Hence, we repeat, the distant Pluto may remain a puzzling object for a long time to come.

58. The Planetesimal Hypothesis Is Probably Right

IF A gas is cooled down below its boiling point, the collisions between its molecules are no longer perfectly elastic. The molecules will join together. Perhaps the gas must be supercooled, in order that droplets will form. On further cooling, instead of liquid droplets, solid crystals will form. We can follow this process with the water in our atmosphere from vapour to rain and snow.

Ter Haar was the first to investigate the process of condensation in the primeval nebula. He proved that the rarefaction of the nebulous matter would not prevent the formation of small droplets and crystals in rather short intervals of time. For this reason we must start from the assumption that several substances in the primeval nebula exist in the liquid or solid state, depending on their kind and distance from the Sun, and hence in the form of planetesimals. These planetesimals are subjected to mutual collisions and hence again to splitting and evaporation. Between planetesimals and the gaseous medium a kind of balance between accretion and dissolution will occur, but to all appearances the condensation to planets will occur via planetesimals. Protoplanets are considered today by almost all investigators as assemblages of planetesimals and not as primarily gaseous globes, with the possible exception of the giants Jupiter and Saturn. They consist probably, for the major part, of the "permanent" gases hydrogen and helium. The planets and even more surely their satellites are of "cold" origin.

For this reason our picture of the revolving solar nebula must undergo some changes. This nebula can hardly be described more truly than as a gas cloud of mainly hydrogen and helium, in which a mass of small crystals extends like a pancake. These "sediments", by accretion, form planetesimals of different size and weight. McCrea and Williams suggest this to be the only way in which light and heavy elements are segregated in the striking manner revealed by the varying composition of satellites and planets, and by the interior of a planet such as our Earth. These authors estimate the average dimension of planetesimals accumulating in a protoplanet at roughly 50 cm, when accumulating in a proto-Moon at roughly 1000 cm. They remark jokingly that: "An Earth exists because a galaxy is slightly dusty."

The present author showed that the non-elastic collisions of the dust particles promote their accretion and further agglomeration, because the gravitational field of the massive centre of every system, primary or secondary, prevents the planetesimals from "escaping". After any collision, these planetesimals are literally swept together in a finite space and consequently urged to collide again and again and lose kinetic energy. Hence "accretional instability" leads to assemblages, waiting for "gravitational instability" to finish the job. The author is even ready to assume, as did also Safronov, that the giant planets were also originally not greater globes, but in fact smaller globes than at present, condensed out of the solid materials mentioned earlier. They may well have acquired most of their hydrogen and helium, because they continued to circulate in a gaseous environment over a long period of time during which this environment slowly disappeared. If this is the true history, the initial masses of the big planets have amounted to the following values in earth masses:

| Jupiter | 41·2 | Uranus | 13·8 |
| Saturn | 29·5 | Neptune | 17·2 |

On the other hand we should, following Öpik, leave open the possibility that solar radiation is absorbed in the relatively dense pancake nebula so effectively that temperatures at distances as large as those of the big planets would permit the existence of solid hydrogen crystals, hydrogen snow, and its entering into these bodies. This might explain why the concentration of helium relative to the concentration of hydrogen in the atmospheres of the giants Jupiter and Saturn is much higher than in the cosmic clouds. The helium, whose freezing point is still lower than the freezing point of hydrogen, remained certainly gaseous throughout the solar system at all times.

59. The Origin of Satellites

THE striking similarity of the satellite systems and the planetary system places beyond any doubt that the secondary systems originated in the same way as the primary system, only on a smaller scale.

The meaning of this conclusion is that the transformation of every planetary ring must have led to a protoplanet consisting of a heavy central body and a light rest mass spinning around it in the form of a flat disk.

One of the main genetical aspects is: although the number of satellites may go into extremes, the dimensions of the systems should be in the same proportion as the masses of their central bodies. This condition is in fact roughly satisfied in all systems.

60. Nature Prefers Even Numbers of Satellites

IMAGINE the existence of two opposite radial density undulations superimposed on the main trend of the density of the primeval disk from the centre to the periphery. The first transformation would lead to the conception of only one major satellite and perhaps of some central and peripheral satellites of negligible mass; the second transformation would lead to the conception of two major satellites and perhaps also of some central and peripheral minor ones.

As in the first case, the density distribution shows maxima where in the second case it shows minima, we may conclude that, when in the first case kinetic energy is gained at the cost of potential energy, the reverse must be true in the second case.

Now it is easily shown that one major satellite could come into existence only by a maximum gain of potential energy on kinetic energy. Since this is a way of development contrary to the natural way, a planet's acquisition of only one satellite is a highly improbable event. On the other hand, the production of two major satellites, associated with a maximum gain of kinetic energy on potential energy, is the most probable event.

This duplication leads easily to further duplications and hence we can draw the remarkable conclusion that even numbers of satellites have a natural advantage over uneven numbers. Now, the four big planets, the four terrestrial planets, the four big satellites of Jupiter and the four big satellites of Uranus teach us that the evolution of four satellites of importance has naturally the greatest probability.

61. Dimensions and Limits of Satellite Systems

IT IS extremely instructive to compare the structure of all satellite systems. In relative measure the system of Mars is the most extensive. Yet the orbits of the two small satellites of Mars, Phobos and Deimos, are so strictly circular and so strictly coincident with the planet's equator that the Martian system must be considered as a perfectly "regular" creation.

How a planet as little as Mars has been able to produce two moons has remained an enigma for a long time. Yet there is no reason whatever to doubt the legitimacy of the children of Mars and no reason to assume, with other investigators, that Mars captured them from the swarm of asteroids. Moreover, the Martian system confirms one of our theoretical conclusions. The development of an even number of satellites is a more probable event than the development of an uneven number. Two satellites is the smallest number to result from the transformation of a nebula in quasi-steady motion. Mars operated with the greatest possible efficiency. Consequently, it is reasonable to consider the orbit of the outer satellite of Mars, Deimos, as the outer limit of any imaginable satellite system. Apparently the gravitational potential of Mars has decreased near Deimos to the minimum value allowing the formation of a secondary.

TABLE 16. OUTER LIMIT OF SATELLITE SYSTEMS EXPRESSED IN PLANET-RADII

Planet	Computed	Outermost satellite	Observed
Mars	7	Deimos	7
Jupiter	1120(600)	VIII, IX, XI, XII	350
Saturn	420	Phoebe	214
Uranus	160	Oberon	24
Neptune	220	—	—

Table 16 is based on this proposition. In some cases, however, critical limits smaller than those given here are added between brackets, since Kuiper showed that satellites circulating at greater distances than the lower of the two limits are in danger. They may be torn away from their system by the Sun or by other planets. In the Jupiter and Saturn families the outermost satellites circulate at a distance which in fact is roughly half the possible distance. In the Uranus family, a relatively wider circle has remained open to satellites. We shall return later to the conditions dominating the evolution of the irregular system of Neptune.

62. Retrograde Satellites

THE peripheral satellites of Jupiter and Saturn in Table 16 are "retrograde" satellites. What should we think of these irregular outer members of some systems? The answer probably is as follows.

The protoplanets originated from rings, and we noted (see section 10) that they will rotate in the "direct" sense, provided the rings are narrow. If, however, ringpieces are united with the protoplanet which have circulated at excessively large or excessively short distances from the Sun, these pieces will show a tendency to move round the planet in the retrograde sense. Now such pieces will, by their very nature, contribute to the formation of outer satellites (Fig. 25). That retrograde satellites occur in the systems of the big planets only, originating from very wide rings, is obvious. As a matter of fact Neptune's heavy satellite Triton is also retrograde. Neptune's system will be considered later. Why Uranus is the only big planet without retrograde satellites is easily understood. This system's exceptional obliquity prevented Uranus from seizing retrograde satellites.

Since secondary nebulae originated as rather extensive flat disks rotating in the direct sense, they will have intercepted here and there a "stray body". Such stray bodies may have moved in the wrong direction and experienced resistance in their planet's nebula. This made them spiral more or less far inward, but also enabled them to collect matter. Retrograde satellites are outsiders, adjoined peripherally and therefore not strictly related to the legitimate members of their families, accumulated out of the disks spinning in the direct sense.

A stray body moving in the right direction may, of course, also be captured, although less easily. Perhaps Hyperion, a remarkably small and irregular satellite of Saturn, is to be considered as a stray body of this kind. Its density is also exceptionally high in proportion to its mass (see section 50).

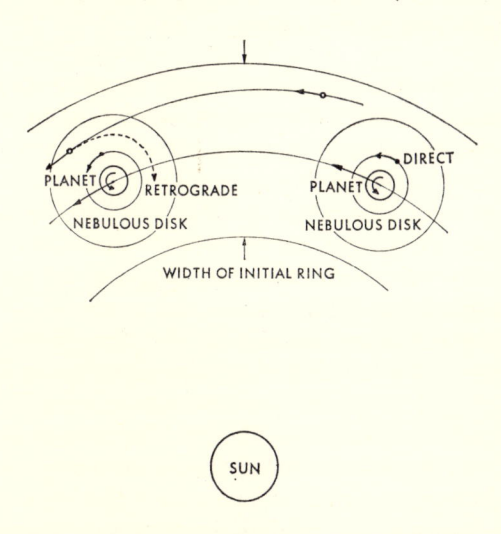

Fig. 25. Picture of the origin of retrograde satellites out of the outer and inner belts of an initial ring that is transformed into a protoplanet.

63. The Two Remaining Great Puzzles

As a matter of fact the origin of the two simplest satellite systems confronts us with the greatest of enigmas; on the one hand, the Earth with its giant satellite Moon, on the other hand, Neptune with its giant retrograde satellite Triton, and that little Nereid, which curiously enough is an outer satellite moving in the direct sense.

64. Earth and Moon

THE history of the Earth–Moon system presents abnormal traits. The mass of the Moon is so large—the 1/81st part of the mass of the Earth—that it causes tidal friction that reduces continuously the speed of the Earth's rotation. The duration of the day increases very slowly, but to an extent just measurable with the aid of the observations of eclipses of the Sun and the Moon made in early historical times.

Fotheringham was able to show that the day is lengthening by 1 sec in almost 100,000 years, while Jeffreys and others could prove that the friction absorbing the energy of the Earth's rotation is for the main part produced by the enormous tidal currents through the Bering Strait. The external friction along the bottom of shallow seas is much stronger than the internal friction in the moving water masses themselves. However, the internal friction in fluids is not negligible. Even if the Earth should not carry oceans the deformation of its "solid" body, due to elasticity and plasticity would cause loss of energy.

A lengthening of the day by 1 sec in 100,000 years is by human standards insignificant, but since the age of our Earth is counted in thousands of millions of years the slowing down of its axial rotation must have been of very great importance in the total course of its evolution. Even during the last 1000 million years, the length of day would have grown by 10,000 sec, or by about 3 hr.

On the other hand, it is very hazardous to calculate this tidal effect by simple extrapolation. We do not know how strong tidal friction was 1000 million years ago. Continents and oceans may have changed shape and many other random events may lie hidden in the past.

If the axial rotation of the Earth is decelerated by lunar tidal forces, the Moon must be accelerated in its orbit round the Earth. This tidal interaction is easily explained. If the forces which the Earth's tidal bulges exert on the Moon are resolved (Fig. 26), we note that the component due to the near tidal bulge in the direction of lunar orbital motion is greater than the component due to the distant tidal bulge in the opposite direction. This difference of attraction explains the "secular acceleration" of lunar motion. The Moon moves in a widening spiral. The Moon is veered out from the Earth.

The end of the process is attained when the period of rotation of the Earth has become equal to the duration of revolution

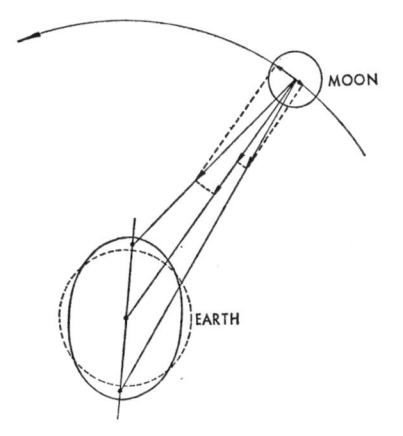

FIG. 26. Acceleration of the orbital motion of the Moon by the tidal forces of the Earth.

of the Moon. Then the day and month are identical while the Earth turns always the same hemisphere towards the Moon, and the two bodies move around their common centre of gravity as if coupled by a solid bar.

The Moon already turns always the same hemisphere towards the Earth. Evidently the deceleration of the rotation of the Moon finished a long time ago, because the Moon is a body much smaller and lighter than the Earth. For the Earth the end of the process lies in the far future.

102 The Origin of the Solar System

The Moon now circulates at a distance from the Earth of 60 earth radii. It will finally recede to a distance of 75 earth radii. At that time the Moon, now revolving around the Earth in 29 days, will revolve around the Earth in 43 days, so one day will be equal to 43 of our present days.

G. H. Darwin was the first to investigate this process of development of the Earth–Moon system. He did so with the utmost care and ingenuity. It is to be remembered, for instance, that the Moon does not move around the Earth in a circular orbit but in a rather eccentric orbit. Secondly, the lunar orbital plane does not coincide with the Earth's equator. Thirdly, the axis of rotation of the Earth is inclined $66° 33'$ to the ecliptic, and finally solar tidal forces should be accounted for. The process is in fact extremely complicated. The position of the axis of rotation of the Earth varies. The Earth moves as a top, a motion known as "precession". The tides vary with these variations and moreover with the distance Moon–Earth. When the Moon stood closer to the Earth the influence of the attraction of the Moon was also greater and changes were more rapid. Last, but not least, how shall we take into account the main geological transformations through which the Earth's crust and the oceans have passed?

G. H. Darwin was able to follow the course of events back to a moment in the past when the Moon moved round the Earth at a shorter distance from the common centre of gravity, in a shorter period and in a more circular orbit than today, while the Moon's orbital plane coincided more closely with the Earth's equator. The Earth then rotated several times more rapidly. This indicates a much more understandable genesis of the Moon. Moreover, Jeffreys proved that the present stretching of the Moon in the direction of the Earth agrees with the deformation to be expected for a globe such as the Moon, when it circulates at a distance of 23 earth radii, unless it were liquid. Hence, our first impression is that the Moon originated at a rather short distance from the Earth and changed from liquid into solid after having receded to a distance of 23 earth radii.

On closer examination this transition must have occurred earlier, because the elasticity and plasticity of the solid moon-body lessens every initial deformation. But serious objections have arisen against the persistence of a lunar "fossil tide". The elasticity and plasticity of even an apparently solid celestial body reach values which simply do not allow internal forces to maintain a fossil tide. What is observed in fact is an unexpected feature of the Moon's internal structure. This is one of the remaining lunar puzzles, but the space age will provide us with the means to solve it before long.

We must now discuss an idea raised by G. H. Darwin; the idea that the Moon once was a part of the Earth and was launched from the Earth at some early date.

Several arguments call for this hypothesis, in particular those from the geomorphological side. The continents gather on one-half of the world, on a hemisphere that has its centre between France and England. The oceans, in particular the Pacific and Indian Oceans together constitute a water hemisphere having its centre near New Zealand. Moreover, the Pacific basin is 600 m deeper than the other oceans and the skin of the Earth, the Sial layer, is thinnest in the Pacific basin. Projects of drilling holes through it are almost ripe for execution. The basaltic layer, the Sima, is not far from naked in the Pacific basin. It is as if a large part of the Earth's upper mantle fails, and this, remarkably enough, on one side of the Earth only. The continents may well have been once united in one primitive continent, Alfred Wegener's "Urcontinent".

For this reason geologists and geophysicists have discussed seriously the question of whether the lost piece of the Earth's crust rests in the Moon. The average density of the Moon, $3 \cdot 3$, is only slightly greater than the density of the terrestrial "sialic" layer, whereas the average density of the whole Earth is $5 \cdot 5$. The Moon, although small compared with the Earth, may well become by compression about 10 per cent greater in density than the lunar materials under normal conditions. If a large piece of the heavier "simatic" layer has been dragged out with it, the Moon would fit not at all badly into the Pacific Ocean.

All this makes the launching of the Moon by the Earth a very tempting supposition, but serious objections have been raised against it.

In the first place, if Moon and Earth were once united the initial body must have rotated around its axis in about 4 hr. Now an Earth–Moon globe rotating with this period, although strongly flattened, would have shown little tendency to fling pieces away. On the other hand, since this propulsion of the Moon from the Earth may have been induced by particular circumstances, it is a good thing to pose the questions: What forms may spinning celestial bodies assume? What are the "equilibrium figures" of spinning liquid masses?

65. Equilibrium Figures of Spinning Liquid Masses

THE equilibrium figure of a spinning liquid mass is determined by the condition that the resultant of gravitational attraction and centrifugal force is perpendicular to this body's surface. The difficulty is that both forces depend on the shape of the body and for their calculation require a knowledge of this shape. The way to a solution therefore is: we look for surfaces that allow the quantities determining their shape to be fixed so that, when density and speed of rotation are given, the equilibrium condition is satisfied.

The dimensions of the body do not matter in this case, because gravitation and centrifugal force remain in the same proportion with varying dimensions of the body, while for the equilibrium only the direction of the resultant of the two forces counts.

MacLaurin, impressed by the well-known figure of Jupiter, was the first to show (1642), that in fact a rotation ellipsoid satisfies the equation of equilibrium of its free surface. There are even, as Simpson was able to show (1743), within a large range of angular velocities two ellipsoids of different degrees of flattening that satisfy the equation. The one is more or less globular, the other more or less lenticular.

It is not for every angular velocity ω that the problem has two solutions. With every given density of the liquid ρ an angular velocity ω_m is associated according to the formula

$$\omega_m^2 : 2\pi\gamma\rho = 0\cdot 225 \qquad (9)$$

in which γ represents the constant of gravitation. If the actual angular velocity ω is less than ω_m there are two rotation ellipsoids satisfying the equation of equilibrium. If ω is greater than ω_m no rotation ellipsoids satisfy the equation of equilibrium. If ω is equal to ω_m there is only one rotation ellipsoid satisfying the equation. The limiting ratio between the polar axis and an equatorial diameter is $1:2\cdot 67$.

Before the quotient $\omega^2:2\pi\gamma\rho$ reaches its maximum value, it has the value

$$\omega^2 : 2\pi\gamma\rho = 0\cdot 187, \qquad (10)$$

a milestone on the way to the development of these spinning bodies. The polar axis and an equatorial diameter are then in the ratio $1:1\cdot 72$. It has been proved that liquid homogeneous spinning rotation ellipsoids, more strongly flattened than this critical model are not "stable" figures. In these cases the smallest deformation causes permanent changes in shape. The given mass, on further cooling and shrinking, cannot remain a rotation ellipsoid.

It was Jacobi who pointed out (1854), that the equation for the free surface of a spinning homogeneous fluid mass is satisfied by a set of non-rotational figures, triaxial ellipsoids. A surprising result, because one would say intuitively that only rotational figures could be equilibrium figures.

A cooling, spinning, liquid globe will thus first assume the shape of a rotation ellipsoid. It gradually becomes more flattened. From the moment that condition (10) is reached the mass assumes the model of a triaxial ellipsoid. Further cooling causes the model to become more and more stretched.

Poincaré showed, however, that the triaxial ellipsoids lose their stability again when

$$\omega^2 : 2\pi\gamma\rho = 0\cdot 142. \qquad (11)$$

The critical figure has axes in the proportion $1 : 1\cdot 25 : 2\cdot 90$ (Fig. 27). The body, after having reached the limiting model of

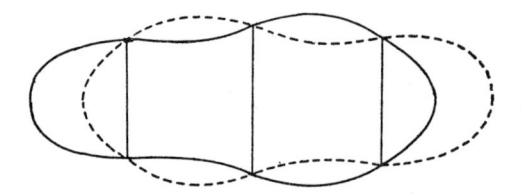

Fig. 27. Transformation of Jacobi's ellipsoid into Poincaré's pear-shaped model.

stable ellipsoids, assumes first an egg shape. This ovoid is subjected to a narrowing that makes it look like a pear. Then, however, according to Liapunov and Jeans, its coherence is threatened. An apioid is unstable from the moment of conception. Further development is catastrophic. The narrow belt grows narrower and finally the pear is split up into two globular bodies of different size.

This theory is valid for homogeneous fluids or gaseous masses. A similar evolution, according to Jeans, is to be expected from unhomogeneous fluid or gaseous masses, provided their structure does not too closely approach that of a heavy nucleus and a light atmosphere. Evidently the evolution of all possible primeval structures leads, on the one hand, to double stars in the simple way just indicated, and, on the other hand, to suns with planetary systems in a way which we are trying to disentangle now.

66. Did Resonance Produce the Moon?

THE fascinating theory of spinning liquid bodies presents possibilities for the splitting of one protoplanet in two parts, Earth and Moon. However, the structure and conditions of rotation of this particular protoplanet can hardly have led to such division by its own forces. Several geophysicists, with G. H. Darwin, have therefore tried to answer the question of whether specific circumstances may have contributed to an expulsion of the Moon by the Earth.

Proto-Earth rotated in a small number of hours, and we have not seriously taken into account the solar tides so far. We know that the solar tides are not half as high as the lunar tides, but yet they must have given proto-Earth the shape of a triaxial ellipsoid. Now it should be remembered that an elastic body, when deformed by external forces, resumes its original shape like a spring as soon as these forces are eliminated. It will even continue to pulsate about its mean dimensions. An apioid will execute pulsations such that humps and hollows change places alternatively (Fig. 28). A pulsation of this kind is shown by a lightly boiled peeled egg. The period of pulsation depends on the type of body. It is called the "proper period" of the body.

Now, every pulsation of an elastic body is amplified when the external force producing the deformation varies with a rhythm equal to the proper period of the body. This phenomenon is called "resonance".

If proto-Earth showed a proper period exactly equal to its

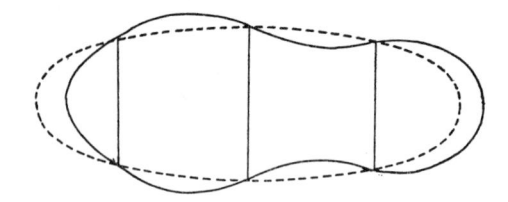

Fig. 28. Pulsations of Poincaré's pear-shaped model inducing its division.

period of rotation, perhaps resonance may have amplified the deformation to such an extent that the splitting up in the apioid manner took place. This is the essence of the "resonance hypothesis" of the origin of Earth and Moon.

It is not impossible that specific circumstances promoted this course of development and the two periods which must have agreed must both have had lengths of some hours. The objections raised by Jeffreys in recent years against the resonance effect are, however, so strong that this hypothesis has been abandoned entirely.

67. Was the Moon Expelled from the Earth?

IN ORDER to split up a protoplanet into Earth and Moon, even if resonance is active, a large amount of energy is required. Hence, the puzzling question remains: What was the source of this energy? A significant quantity of potential energy was liberated, as Wise pointed out, when the Earth's core was concentrated, but this can hardly have contributed significantly to the Moon's expulsion.

There are several more arguments against a separation of Earth and Moon. If the splitting up of a celestial body should occur in the way considered by Poincaré, the proportion between the masses of the smaller and the larger body has to remain near one-third. The reason for this is Roche's limit, which allows a secondary body to stay safely in the field of force of the primary body only when its mass is large enough. The actual proportion of the masses of Moon and Earth is 1/81st. How could so small a part of the Earth's mass be launched without being destroyed? The density of the Moon is $3 \cdot 3$ whereas the density of the Earth is $5 \cdot 5$. Consequently the Moon cannot come closer to the Earth than 3 earth radii without being in danger. Hence, the Moon can never have circulated round the Earth at shorter distance than 3 earth radii.

If in fact the Moon was separated from the Earth it must have been launched immediately beyond 3 earth radii. Now, an event of this kind is not excluded. Physical and chemical forces capable of propelling a body like our Moon are available in our Earth, but even so the difficulties are not overcome. If a missile leaves the Earth it flies away in an elliptic or in a hyperbolic orbit. In the first case it drops back on Earth. In the second case it flies away into interplanetary space. It may start moving as an independent little planet round the Sun, but it will not start moving in a closed orbit round the Earth as the Moon must have done.

In our space age, in order to make a future satellite depart from the Earth, we have to launch a secondary rocket from a primary one. A natural event of this kind would require such improbable conditions that one can reasonably discard it. One possibility remains: the Moon was destroyed in the beginning and remained circulating round the Earth as a ring of particulate matter like Saturn's ring. Why, then, assume that the Moon was expelled from the Earth? In this case the origin of the Moon might well have been "normal", as the condensation product of a dust ring which circulated outside the zone of danger.

68. Did the Earth Capture the Moon?

THERE are quite a number of theories based on this hypothesis of the Moon's origin, although every student of the subject realizes how hopelessly improbable the capture of a satellite by a planet is, in particular when the satellite is as massive as our Moon, and when it is moving in the "direct" sense round its primary.

One capture theory, however, has received serious attention, viz. Gerstenkorn's revision and extension of Darwin's tidal theory of the Moon's history. It is strongly supported by MacDonald. Gerstenkorn, with the aid of electronic computers showed that the Moon, originally an independent small planet, was probably transferred by the Earth into its gravity field in an early phase of the evolution of our system.

The Moon started its career as a "retrograde" satellite of the Earth. Retrograde satellites by tidal interaction approach their "parent planets". Thus the Moon, after having been captured, came gradually nearer to the Earth. Tidal forces equalized the periods of the Earth's rotation and the Moon's revolution, while the Moon reached a minimum distance from the Earth of $2 \cdot 89$ earth radii. Part of our initial satellite dropped on Earth whereas the other part, the Moon, veered out from the Earth.

Hence capture apparently confronts our big satellite with the same danger as does expulsion. It has to emerge safely from just inside Roche's limit.

Now let us not lose sight of the fact that the origin of the Moon is only one particular aspect of the problem of the origin of satellites in general. We are hardly going to profit by hypotheses *ad hoc* for a special case, when we have not yet investigated if the special case is not derivable in a logical way from the general case.

69. Was the Moon Perhaps a Normal Satellite?

THE author conceded that the production by a planet of only one satellite was a most improbable event. For this reason our Earth was to be regarded with suspicion. Now this suspicion was cherished by the advocates of the two theories mentioned so far, the expulsion theory and the capture theory of the Moon. What is our logical inference? The evolution of the Moon must have been paralleled by the evolution of one other satellite of significant mass. When this problem is analysed numerically we are strongly persuaded that the inner satellite, gravitating towards the centre by loss of energy due to viscosity, was condensed on the Earth whereas the Moon is that second outer satellite.

Öpik and the author, along completely different lines of reasoning, reached the same conclusion. The Moon originated probably at a distance of 5·8 earth radii. A third satellite originated at a distance of $5 \cdot 8^2$ or 34 earth radii. This is quite in accordance with our previous conclusion that the Earth's system, in conformity with the Martian system, should have been able to produce a peripheral satellite at a distance of, but no more than, 35 earth radii.

The annular embryo of this latter satellite undoubtedly never condensed into one body. Its agglomeration resulted in a large number of planetesimals. These planetesimals are likely to have bombarded the Moon, creating its "maria" and many impact craters when the Moon, receding by tidal action, passed the distance of 34 earth radii. Such an origin of the major part of lunar features was first suggested by Kuiper.

The ratio of the mass of the Moon m_m and of the total mass m_e of the material of the disk circulating between the Earth's equator and the distance of separation between the two main rings, is

$$\frac{m_m}{m_e} = 0 \cdot 76. \tag{12}$$

Whereas the mass of the Moon amounts to 0·0123 earth masses, the mass of the failing satellite would have amounted to 0·0162 earth masses. The total mass of the planetesimals circulating initially round the Earth would have amounted to roughly 0·03 earth masses, in excellent agreement with the swarm of bodies of total mass 0·01– 0·1 earth masses, which, according to Ruskol, might have formed about the Earth during its period of growth.

The ratio of the total mass of the peripheral belt of planetesimals m_p and the mass of the Moon is

$$\frac{m_p}{m_m} = 0 \cdot 00058. \tag{13}$$

This is a numerically interesting conclusion. Urey estimated the diameter of the planetesimal, the largest of all, which generated the Mare Imbrium, at 230 km. The diameter of the Moon is 3476 km. If the density of this planetesimal is assumed to be equal to the density of the Moon, the ratio of the masses of the two bodies is

$$\frac{\text{Mare Imbrium planetesimal}}{\text{Moon}} = 0 \cdot 00048. \tag{14}$$

This particular mass is in excellent agreement with the total mass of the planetesimals given by (13).

Let us terminate the discussion of the terrestrial system by computing the duration of revolution of the Moon at its birth. It was 19·4 hr. The day counted roughly no more than 6·5 hr. On the other hand, the Earth apparently did not rotate at all in its earliest state when the dust ring providing for the inner satellite was still spinning round it. This, however, may well be considered as a logical consequence of the strong tidal friction which must have operated during the time when the primeval Earth was sufficiently fluid to permit the concentration of its iron–nickel core. Venus and Mercury are still in this condition.

70. Neptune and its Satellites

ANOTHER singular case is that of Neptune and its satellites. Neptune, according to the rules, is spinning in the direct sense and possesses a very small satellite, Nereid, discovered by Kuiper. This satellite is moving around the planet at a great distance, also in the direct sense, although its orbit is considerably eccentric.

A most remarkable fact, however, is that Neptune possesses a very heavy satellite, Triton, moving at a mean distance of 13·3 planet radii in an almost circular orbit, and in the retrograde sense.

The systems of Jupiter and Saturn both contain a few very small retrograde satellites moving along the periphery of these systems. We recognized them as outsiders having entered the initial dust disks surrounding their planet. Neptune very probably once also possessed a dust disk, rotating in the direct sense. This dust disk might have produced a number of regular satellites if a massive satellite had not penetrated into the disk from the reverse direction and remained caught like a fly in a spider's web (Fig. 29).

If Triton had not experienced resistance in Neptune's dust disk, it would probably have moved out again from Neptune's field of attraction. The resistance transformed Triton's hyperbolic orbit relative to Neptune into an elliptic one. The way in which this resistance acts has been studied, as was noted earlier, by Nölke. The body assembles dust from the disk. Its orbit shrinks, becoming less and less eccentric, and less and less inclined to the equatorial plane of the planet, which, we may assume, coincides with the plane of symmetry of the dust disk.

Thus Triton came gradually closer to the planet, meanwhile consuming the dust disk. This results surprisingly in a relatively heavy satellite in retrograde motion at a relatively short distance from the planet. We might even suppose that Triton's

114 The Origin of the Solar System

history has not yet ended, because what happened to Triton may have been the reverse of what happened to the Moon. A satellite moving in the opposite direction to the planet's rotation approaches the planet as a result of tidal interaction,

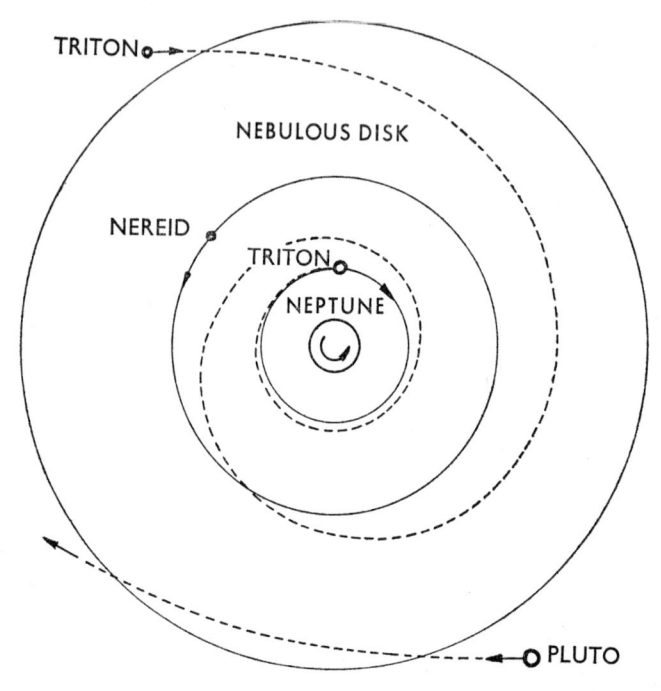

FIG. 29. What may have occurred around Neptune. Capture of retrograde Triton and freedom allowed to Pluto. The speed of Triton's approach to Neptune is greatly exaggerated.

whereas the Moon moved away from the Earth. Some time in the far future Triton may therefore crash into Neptune.

Table 16 shows that Neptune might have possessed satellites up to a distance of 220 planet radii from the centre. Its initial dust disk may well have extended so far.

It is therefore not in the least improbable that Triton approached Neptune from a distance of more than 100 planet radii. Its present distance is 13·3 planet radii. In the course of this evolution Triton must have crossed Nereid's orbit. At that time Triton perturbed Nereid. This may explain the large eccentricity of Nereid's orbit. It is not less than 0·76. The present shortest distance of Nereid from Neptune is 55 planet radii. Probably Nereid moved in a plane nearly coincident with the equatorial plane of the planet, in a nearly circular orbit, this having a radius of, perhaps, 60 planet radii. This is a very reasonable distance for a small satellite moving in the direct sense at the periphery of a satellite system.

Triton's crossing of Neptune's system must have completely prevented the development of regular satellites. For reasons mentioned earlier, the author is inclined to assume that Neptune would have produced four major satellites, had Triton not intervened and claimed the available building materials for its own use.

If it is assumed that Triton initially circulated at a distance from the centre nine times as great as it does today, that is at a distance of 120 planet radii, we can prove that Triton must have assembled a two-fifths part of its present mass in the course of its approach to Neptune. This part of its mass, or the 1/2000th part of Neptune's mass, must therefore have constituted the mass of the dust disk initially rotating around Neptune. If four regular satellites have been formed out of this mass, each of them would have obtained a mass of about the 1/8000th part of Neptune's mass. This proportion is in excellent agreement with the normal proportion in the other satellite systems.

71. The Question of Pluto

WE EARLIER expressed our surprise that from the large dust disk out of which the planets condensed, the extremely rarified peripheral zone outside Neptune's ring should have given birth to a planet. Moreover, this planet moves around the Sun in an orbit of such eccentricity (Table 1) that its perihelion is inside Neptune's orbit.

It is really remarkable that the planet Pluto and the satellite Triton are so similar. This fact induced several investigators to postulate their common origin. Opinions went in two directions. Lyttleton assumed that Triton and Pluto had been twin satellites of Neptune, both circulating in the sense of rotation of the planet. At a certain time Triton and Pluto came very near each other. At this meeting Triton reversed its direction of motion, whereas Pluto was expelled from Neptune's system. An event like this, however, seems very improbable.

The opposite event is more likely. Triton and Pluto were originally two independent little planets, near neighbours of Neptune. At some stage Neptune captured Triton. This supposition was made by Dauvillier and Camichel. The capture of Triton was greatly simplified, if Triton experienced the resistance of Neptune's dust disk. For this reason the author considers a variation on the present theme as the more probable event. Triton and Pluto were condensation products of the outermost and innermost belts of the large dust ring from which Neptune originated. We know that these belts may produce retrograde satellites. Triton was captured, Pluto was not captured and having passed near Neptune, regained liberty and moved away in space as an independent planet.

However, whether Pluto's behaviour was dependent on Neptune to any significant extent has become uncertain. Cohen and Hubbard pointed out that Pluto is safe from close encounters with Neptune. No meetings occur nearer than 18 a.u., and hence the thesis that Pluto was an independent planet by birth has regained plausibility.

72. The Systems of Jupiter, Saturn, and Uranus as Family Portraits

WE ARE now leaving the satellite systems with one or two members in order to make a comparison between the systems with numerous satellites. The systems of Jupiter and Uranus, as are shown by Table 17, are so similar that one is induced to ask whether these two are not *the* classical examples of satellite systems.

TABLE 17. TWO SIMILAR SATELLITE SYSTEMS

Jupiter	Uranus
V.	Miranda
I. Io	Ariel
II. Europa	Umbriel
III. Ganymede	Titania
IV. Callisto	Oberon
VI, VII, X retrograde VIII, IX, XI, XII	?

The innermost satellite is small. Then follow four big satellites. Further outwards Jupiter possesses a triplet of small satellites, circulating in the direct sense, and still further outwards a quadruplet of retrograde small satellites. O. Struve found indications of the existence of a faint ring fitting closely around Jupiter.

As was pointed out before, we can hardly expect retrograde satellites of Uranus, but a small satellite or some small satellites, corresponding with the numbers VI, VII, and X of Jupiter, may yet be found.

How is the great number of satellites in Saturn's system to be grouped between the two systems just mentioned? In order to understand this correctly we may have to treat Saturn's system independently in the same way as was done with the planetary system. The reliability of this treatment rests on the fact that the masses of Saturn's satellites have been determined very accurately from perturbations. The values found by G. Struve are summarized in Table 18. The mass of Saturn's tenth satellite, Janus, recently discovered by Dollfus, is not yet given.

TABLE 18. THE MASSES OF SATURN'S SATELLITES EXPRESSED AS A FRACTION OF THE PLANET'S MASS

Mimas	1:14,960,000
Enceladus	6,622,000
Thetys	876,000
Dione	541,000
Rhea	250,000
Titan	4033
Hyperion	5,000,000
Japetus	375,000

Now, because the ring of asteroids has to be counted among the planets and reasons were given for an account of three virtual planets inside Mercury's orbit, we are obliged to count Saturn's ring among its satellites. There is every reason to count the ring not as one satellite but as two satellites. The ring is in fact divided into three specific zones, A, B, and C (Fig. 18). The central one is the veil ring C, further outwards follow two bright rings, B and A, separated by the Cassini division. However, the Cassini division may be explained by perturbations. A small satellite when circulating through this division would be thrown permanently out of its orbit, because the periods of revolution of Mimas and the small satellite here suggested are in the proportion 1:2 exactly. The Cassini division is a "resonance gap". Such characteristic circumstances are not at all in contradiction with the supposed process of origin of secondary systems. Several outstanding relations between the periods of revolution of the satellites of Saturn have been pointed out, and the same is true of the satellites of Jupiter. These relations may well be considered as the normal and perhaps even basic results of the processes associated with the creation of systems of secondaries. But let us count the two bright rings *A* and *B* as one unfinished satellite.

The best results of a computation of the masses of the satellites of Saturn, made on the basis of the same formula as was applied when the masses of the planets were approximated, are given in Table 19.

TABLE 19. THE MASSES OF SATURN'S SATELLITES ACCORDING TO THEORY AND OBSERVATION

| | Logarithm of distance (radius of planet = 1) || Logarithm of mass (mass of planet = 1) ||
	Observed	Assumed	Computed	Observed
Equator	0	0		
Mean ring *C*	0·110	0·118	−6·78	
Mean ring *B–A*	0·220	0·236	−6·42	
Janus	0·324	0·354	−6·62	
Mimas	0·487	0·472	−7·16	−7·17
Enceladus	0·595	0·590	−6·83	−6·82
Thetys	0·688	0·708	−5·98	−5·94
Dione	0·795	0·826	−5·51	−5·73
Rhea	0·940	0·944	−5·50	−5·40
		1·062	−5·25 ⎫	
		1·180	−4·33 ⎪	
Titan	1·306	1·296	−3·95 ⎬ 3·70	−3·61
Hyperion	1·397	1·416	−4·48 ⎪	−6·70
		1·534	−5·30 ⎭	
		1·652	−5·83 ⎫	
Japetus	1·770	1·770	−5·83 ⎬ −5·51	−5·57
		1·888	−6·73 ⎭	

Table 19 does not include the retrograde satellite Phoebe. Hyperion, too, shows definitely abnormal properties. Apparently its density is so high that we might prefer to consider Hyperion as a planetoid invader into the system of Saturn. If Hyperion is dropped, Table 19 requires some explanation of what happened in the cases of Titan and Japetus. The relatively large weights of these satellites, associated with the occupation of several terms in the geometric series of orbit radii, are rather convincing evidence that materials of the disk ready to form five satellites were united in Titan, whereas the materials ready to form three satellites were united in Japetus. Events such as these may be expected to occur, in particular in a case like this, when an exceptionally great number of rings were on the point of agglomeration. Those who have become acquainted with the work of Belot will recognize in Table 19 a scheme already discussed by him.

Important estimates are those of the unknown masses of Saturn's innermost satellite Janus and of its rings. These masses when expressed in the planet's mass as a unit, have the following values:

$$\text{Janus} = 1 : 4,200,000$$
$$\text{main ring } A \text{ and } B = 1 : 2,600,000$$
$$\text{veil ring } C = 1 : 6,000,000$$

These values are reasonable, since the bright rings have the greatest and the veil ring the smallest mass, whereas the total mass, viz. 1:1,200,000, appears to be of the right order of magnitude. Recent observations would suggest that part of the matter available to form Janus was shifted to the bright rings.

There is no reason for a dust ring inside ring C, because the radius of this ring would have been equal with the radius of the planet's equator. At the other end, the outermost satellite moving in the direct sense, Japetus, behaves irregularly. Its orbit is strongly inclined to the equator of the planet. This makes the discovery of some regular satellite between Japetus and the retrograde Phoebe extremely improbable. Therefore, apart from the melting together of several "protosatellites" the whole series of satellites of Saturn is strikingly complete.

73. Comparative Anatomy of all Satellite Systems

ARGUMENTS were given for the thesis that a planet's possession of an even number of satellites is more probable than the possession of an odd number. The possession of only one satellite, as in the case of Earth and Moon, requires, therefore, the introduction of a virtual second satellite. Let us call it Lucifer, as it would have fallen to the Earth.

We concluded that the ratio between the orbital radii of Lucifer and the Moon was $5 \cdot 8$, or $\log r_{n+1} - \log r_n = 0 \cdot 77$. The ratio between the orbital radii of the two Martian satellites Deimos and Phobos is $6 \cdot 9 : 2 \cdot 8 = 2 \cdot 5$, or $\log r_{n+1} - \log r_n = 0 \cdot 40$. These proportions seem relatively high when compared with those in the numerous systems. However, the evolution of a satellite system with four big members apparently results from a duplication of a system with only two members. In such cases four main rings in the place of two have been produced. Therewith $\log r_{n+1} - \log r_n = 0 \cdot 20$ should have resulted. As a matter of fact we find $\log r_{n+1} - \log r_n = 0 \cdot 22$ and $\log r_{n+1} - \log r_n = 0 \cdot 17$ in the systems of Jupiter and Uranus respectively. The next duplication would lead theoretically to $\log r_{n+1} - \log r_n = 0 \cdot 10$, whereas $\log r_{n+1} - \log r_n = 0 \cdot 12$ is realized in the system of Saturn. This is a very promising aspect of the theory of planetary evolution.

Now, Saturn possesses nine regular satellites. However, with its two rings and five "unfinished" satellites, Saturn's system involves sixteen members "potentially". In this case a further duplication was apparently due to occur. It is, however, more reasonable to attack the problem from the other end and to

122   The Origin of the Solar System

consider the system of Saturn as involving sixteen possible members, including eight major ones, and descend from this elaborate system to the systems of eight possible members, with four major ones, such as those of Jupiter and Uranus, and finally to the systems with about four possible members, with two major ones, those of the Earth and Mars.

A survey from this point of view, of the origin of all known satellites and the secular motions of two of them is given in Table 20. The symmetry and logic of the scheme strongly supports the hypothesis developed here. Again, the existence of one or more small satellites of Uranus circulating in the direct sense beyond Oberon, seems to possess a high degree of probability.

An interesting result, not yet mentioned, but particularly instructive, is the rule that the Bode ratio, viz. the value $\log r_{n+1} - \log r_n$ in all systems is gradually increasing with the average density ρ of the central body;

	$\bar{\rho}$	$\log r_{n+1} - \log r_n$
Earth	5·52	0·77
Mars	4·12	0·40
Neptune	2·47	?
Uranus	1·56	0·17
Jupiter	1·35	0·22
Saturn	0·71	0·12

Neptune in the third column bears a question mark, but who would object to the supposition that the satellite system of Neptune, if retrograde Triton had not destroyed it, would have been distinguished by a value $\log r_{n+1} - \log r_n$, roughly 0·3?

The value of this relationship can hardly be overestimated. It suggests a singular position of Saturn in the evolution of the solar system. Perhaps Saturn, not Jupiter, was the first-born planet, while the other planets have been created in succession starting from Saturn both inwards and outwards.

TABLE 20. THE SCHEME OF SATELLITE SYSTEMS, SUPPOSED COMPLETE

Earth						Moon(f) 3·84
Mars					III 2·14	
Jupiter	V 1·8	Io 4·2	Eu 6·7		VI, VII, X 117	retrograde VIII, IX, XI, XII 235
Saturn Rings 0·7–1·4	Ja Mi 1·6 1·9	En Th 2·4 3·0	Di Rh 3·8 5·3	Ti 12·2	* Ja * 35·6 ?	Ph 129
Uranus	Mi 1·2	Ar 1·9	Um 2·7			
Neptune		*	* Tr(f) 3·6		Ne 16	←Tr(s) 30

Moon(s)→ 0·37
De 0·24
Ga 10·7 * *
Ti 4·4 *
Ca 18·8 * *
Ob 5·9 *

(s) = start; (f) = finish; * = virtual; ? = probably existing.
The numbers below the initials of the satellites give the semi-major axes of the satellite orbits, expressed in 10^{10} cm.

74. Why not Satellites of Satellites?

IN REPLY to this obvious question it can be ascertained that not one satellite could have acquired satellites of a lower order. We can prove this indirectly with the aid of the ratio which must have existed between the values of the gravitational potential of the central bodies and the dimensions of their dust disks. The small Mars, as we know, just managed to obtain satellites. Deimos, the most hazardous case for Mars, circulates at a distance of 7 planet radii from the centre. Figure 23 shows that the heaviest satellites, Titan of Saturn and Ganymede of Jupiter, have masses equal to about one-quarter Mars mass. Their density, however, is as $2 \cdot 4$ against $4 \cdot 1$, the density of Mars. The radii of these satellites are consequently only $1 \cdot 3$ times smaller than the radius of Mars. The value of the gravitational potential that Mars exerts near Deimos, is the same as the value found for Titan and Ganymede at a distance of $2 \cdot 3$ satellite radii. This distance is already inside the Roche danger zone. When considering satellites of successively smaller dimensions, we see that very soon this value of the gravitational potential is no longer reached outside the surface of the satellite. In all these cases secondary satellites are excluded. Only Titan and Ganymede might possess rings of meteorites.

Some relationship must exist between the factors which have prevented the smaller members of our solar system from producing secondaries and the factors associated with their lack of an atmosphere. The nebulous disks, in quasi-steady motion because of internal friction, which precede the formation of secondaries, are essentially a kind of atmosphere, only abnormally flat and extended. It is therefore certainly not by chance that Titan, at the threshold of possessing second-order satellites, is the only satellite with a very light atmosphere of methane gas, as observed by Kuiper.

75. A Few Words About our Home in the Solar System

THROUGH what temperature range has the Earth gone?

Present temperatures in the Earth's interior, on the basis of different arguments, are estimated not to exceed 4–5000°C absolute. In the course of thousands of millions of years of geological history, temperatures in the Earth's interior cannot have decreased significantly. Its conductive power is very low. Yet, at one time, circumstances must have been such as to induce molten iron to sink to the centre of the Earth. The iron must have lost therewith the oxygen with which it was chemically bound during its original dispersion in the primeval nebula.

Urey estimates the temperature of the Earth in this stage at 2000°C absolute. During the final differentiation of our globe, whatever came floating to the surface was cooled by depression, whatever sank down was heated by compression. Thus originated the fluid iron and nickel earthcore and the solid stone earthmantle. These exist today almost unchanged. A small inner core formed under extremely high pressure, while the Earth's crust cooled down rather quickly to its present temperature.

However, the heat that counteracted the cooling of the Earth since its creation must have been that developed by its radioactive constituents. The most important of these are the rare, but rather intensively radioactive uranium and thorium, and the abundant, but radioactively much weaker potassium, whose "isotope", atomic weight 40, changes slowly into argon.

These radioactive substances, during the period of intense convection that must have characterized the Earth for a long time, apparently accumulated almost exclusively in the Earth's crust. They seem to avoid close packings. In fact, if they had been accumulated in the interior of the globe in the same concentration, the Earth would have become hotter than it is now.

It is equally surprising that we do not know whether our world at the present time is growing warmer or colder.

Sea and air could never have stood the 2000°C absolute just mentioned, for they would have evaporated from the Earth. This must indeed have happened to the inert gas neon, because it is much rarer on Earth than might have been expected from cosmic composition. Moreover, geology has not taught us anything about the condensation at 100°C of a very heavy primary atmosphere, consisting almost entirely of water vapour. Hydrosphere and atmosphere most probably have been sweated out of the Earth in an early cool stage.

Where all this water has been stowed away is an interesting problem. The assumption that part of the water on the Earth is of meteoritic origin should not be discarded too easily. The author entertains the idea that the inner satellite, the one that only existed in the ring phase and covered the Earth, has contributed a great deal to the oceans.

Our present geophysical relations with the outer satellite, the Moon, include the rare occurrence of impacts of swarms of "tektites", a glassy kind of meteorite found dispersed over a few extensive areas on Earth, the main one being South-east Asia, the Philippines, Indonesia, and Australia. Almost all investigators are agreed that tektites are small pieces of the lunar surface, propelled from the Moon when it is hit by a heavy normal meteorite.

Not only the naked lunar surface, but also the Earth's crust shows the signs of meteoritic impacts. However, erosion acts so strongly in our terrestrial environment that only the largest impact craters, such as the famous Arizona crater, still exhibit their cosmic origin (Plate V).

Bibliography

ALFVÉN, H. (1954) *On the Origin of the Solar System*, Clarendon Press, Oxford.

BATES, D. R. (1957) (Editor) *The Planet Earth*, Pergamon Press, London.

CHAMBERLIN, T. C. (1927) *The Origin of the Earth*, University of Chicago Science Series.

FISHER, C. (1945) *The Story of the Moon*, Doubleday, Doran & Co., New York.

GAMOW, G. (1959) *Biography of the Earth*, revised edition, Macmillan, London.

HOYLE, F. (1955) *Frontiers of Astronomy*, Heinemann, London.

JEFFREYS, H. (1924) *The Earth, its Origin, History and Physical Constitution*, Cambridge University Press.

KUIPER, G. P. (1956) The formation of the planets, *Journal Royal Astronomical Society Canada*, vol. 50.

RUSSELL, H. N. (1935) *The Solar System and its Origin*, Macmillan, New York.

SCHMIDT, O. J. (1958) *A Theory of Earth's Origin*, Foreign Languages Publishing House, Moscow.

TER HAAR, D. (1946) *Studies of the Origin of the Solar System*, Kgl. Danske Videnskabernes Selskab, Copenhagen.

UREY, H. C. (1952) *The Planets: Their Origin and Development*, Oxford University Press.

Author Index

Alfven, H. 33, 34, 52
Arrhenius, Sv. 21

Belot, E. 120
Berlage, H. P. 40, 47, 54, 67, 74, 85, 94, 111, 121, 124
Birkeland, R. 33, 34
Bode, J. E. 4, 5, 23, 69, 122
Brouwer, D. 58
Brown, H. 51
Buffon, G. L. L. 21

Camichel, H. 116
Cassini, G. D. 59, 60, 118
Chamberlin, T. C. 20, 23, 58
Chandrasekhar, S. 42
Coehn, C. J. 116

Darwin, G. H. 102, 103, 107
Dauvillier, A. 31, 33, 116
Descartes, R. 10, 11
Dollfus, A. 118

Eddington, A. S. 26

Fotheringham, J. K. 100

Gerasimović, B. 38
Gerstenkorn, H. 110

Halley, E. 81
Halm, J. 17
Heisenberg, W. 42
Helmholtz, H. 35
Herschel, F. W. 11
Hirayama, K. 58
Hoyle, F. 29, 31, 61
Hubbard, E. C. 116
Hubble, E. 27
Huygens, Chr. 11

Jacobi, C. G. J. 66, 105
Jeans, J. H. 18, 23, 25, 27, 28, 31, 106
Jeffreys, H. 27, 28, 46, 100, 102, 108

Kant, I. 11, 14, 20, 47
Kepler, J. 4, 17, 38, 63
Kolmogorov, A. N. 42
Korteweg, D. J. 35
Kothari, D. S. 49
Kuiper, G. P. 7, 47, 51, 52, 53, 59, 71, 91, 97, 111, 113, 124

Lagrange, J. L. 18
Laplace, P. S. 14, 15, 16, 20, 25, 46
Lemaître, G. 26
Liapunov, A. M. 106
Lighthill, M. J. 80
Lüst, R. 34, 39, 52
Lyttleton, R. A. 29, 31, 116

MacDonald, G. J. F. 110
MacLaurin 105
McCrea, W. H. 94
Moulton, F. R. 22, 23, 58

Newton, I. 11, 36
Nölke, F. 28, 46, 113

Oort, J. H. 22, 82
Öpik, E. J. 49, 94, 111

Poincaré, H. 18, 20, 66, 106, 109
Poynting, H. P. 83

Ramsey, W. H. 80
Rayleigh, Lord 35
Robertson, H. P. 83
Roche, E. 59, 91, 124
Ruskol, E. L. 112
Russell, H. N. 50

Safronov, V. S. 46, 94
Schlüter, H. 34, 52
Schmidt, O. J. 67
Simpson, 105
Sitter, W. de 75
Strömgren, B. 81
Struve, G. 75, 118
Struve, O. 18

Ter Haar, D. 51, 57, 71, 93
Titius 4, 5, 23, 69
Tuominen, J. 46

Urey, H. C. 58, 80, 112, 125

Wegener, A. 103
Weizsäcker, C. F. von 29, 39, 42, 45, 46, 47, 52, 53, 85
Whipple, F. L. 81, 84
Williams, J. P. 94
Wise, D. U. 108
Woolfson, M. M. 25